I am honored to dedicate this book to my father, Jason Minick, for his presence in my life and for teaching me through example how to live, love, and simply be. I am thankful for his insight, support, direction, and for all he added to my life.

FUEL UP

FUEL UP

Using the Principles of Sports Nutrition to Train Like a Pro

**By Eric Sternlicht, Ph.D.,
with Neil Feineman**

A Perigee Book

A Perigee Book
Published by The Berkley Publishing Group
A division of Penguin Putnam Inc.
375 Hudson Street
New York, New York 10014

Copyright © 2001 by Eric Sternlicht, Ph.D.
Information on nutritive values for selected foods found on pp. 233–255 from
Bowes & Church's Food Values of Portions Commonly Used, Sixteenth Edition by
Jean A. T. Pennington, 1994, J. B. Lippincott Co., used by permission of
Lippincott Williams & Wilkins.
Book design by Tiffany Kukec
Cover design by Liz Sheehan
Cover photo of woman drinking water by J. Silver/Superstock
Cover photo of man using dumbbells by J. Silver/Superstock
Cover photo of woman stretching by Roger Allyn Lee/Superstock

First edition: January 2002

Published simultaneously in Canada.

Visit our website at www.penguinputnam.com

Library of Congress Cataloging-in-Publication Data

Sternlicht, Eric.
    Fuel up : using the principles of sports nutrition to train like a pro / Eric Sternlicht, with Neil Feineman.
        p. cm.
    Includes index.
    ISBN 0-399-52742-7
    1. Athletes—Nutrition. I. Feineman, Neil. II. Title.

TX361.A8 S74 2002
613.2'024'796—dc21

2001133071

PRINTED IN THE UNITED STATES OF AMERICA

10 9 8 7 6 5 4 3 2 1

Contents

Acknowledgments

I would like to thank all those people who have helped shape my life and those who have influenced me in my chosen profession:

The many teachers and professors I had over the years. In particular I want to thank Roland Roy, Ph.D., the Human Physiology professor who sparked my interest in the human body and how it works. My graduate advisor, R. James Barnard, Ph.D., along with Brian Whipp, Ph.D., and V. Reggie Edgerton, Ph.D., for sharing their knowledge, style, and enthusiasm for the fields of science and medicine. And finally, Glen Grimditch, Ph.D., fellow doctoral student and colleague with whom I started my nutrition and exercise consulting company, Simply Fit.

The numerous editors and publishers of the various magazines I've written for over the years for giving me the opportunity to hone my writing skills and for being able to share the scientific information I've come across with a much larger and varied audience than the students or clients I've worked with.

Those clients in the entertainment industry, athletic arena, and the general public who have trusted me and benefited from the knowledge I have shared with them. In particular, I want to thank Steve Hegg, who along with myself, put the principles contained in this book into practice with great success.

My friends and mentors who are too numerous to mention by name but who include Scott, Mona, Barry, Paul, Eric, Mark, Joel, Larry, and Israel. Special thanks goes to my department chair, colleague, coresearcher, and close friend, Stuart Rugg, Ph.D., for not only reading this manuscript in various forms, but also for accommodating my unorthodox schedule and consulting work throughout the years.

My agent, Neeti Madan, for believing in me and this project and my editor, Sheila Curry Oakes, for her assistance in polishing this book into the one you're reading today. I also want to thank Samantha Dunn for her help in creating a proposal for this book that would entice Neeti to take the project on.

I am especially thankful to my coauthor, Neil, who has become a valued friend and mentor over the years and a wonderful collaborator. He makes working a pleasure, and I feel fortunate to have someone so talented and gifted to share this project with.

Finally, I want to thank my family, in particular my loving, involved, and supportive wife, Christy, and our beautiful daughter, Elena. They add so much to my life and I am forever thankful for their presence and continued support.

Introduction

ON A PERSONAL NOTE

Athletics always came naturally to me: I was skiing by the time I was four, competed as a swimmer when I was seven, lettered in soccer in high school, and walked away from a professional ski career when I was 18 so I could go to college.

While at the University of California at Los Angeles, I got drawn into the worlds of physiology and competitive bodybuilding. That gave me access to the best of both worlds. I worked with accomplished academicians in a traditional setting and with professional bodybuilders in the gym. I competed in state and regional competitions for the next eight years, winning the Collegiate Mr. America contest. Some colleagues thought I was odd to want to be so big, but I loved using bodybuilding as an escape from the rigors of studying for my masters and doctorate degrees.

In 1985, I put my scientific and practical expertise to work by founding my own consulting business, Simply Fit. Although I initially planned on working with athletes and the general public, my academic credentials and athletic look gave me credibility with the entertainment industry. Before long, I had consulted for entertainers such as Clint Eastwood, Lou Ferrigno, and Deborah Shelton so they could get into shape for the camera.

I continued to train entertainers and professional athletes and work as a consultant to corporations such as Disney, Sony, and ESPN. In 1991, I got my biggest corporate job up to that point, developing the Slide Reebok Training Program. I had to oversee complicated research, write manuals and videos about the slideboard, and travel extensively to promote the program. It was a full-time job, and was complicated by the fact that I was also teaching at two colleges, doing guest spots on television shows such as ESPN's *Body Shaping*, and cycling competitively.

Although I was promoting health and fitness, I had neglected to take most of my own advice. I was tired and run-down from work both at home and on the road, the stress of travel, and a full-time training load. I knew I needed to cut back on something, but I enjoyed everything I was involved with and couldn't decide what to give up. I was out of balance but thought I could juggle the load for just a little longer.

Then, after a business trip to Spain, I became very ill. We suspected I was infected with an intestinal parasite and, after the tests came back negative, Epstein-Barr Syndrome. In any case, my body shut down for months. Because I had been so fit before I became ill, I could function at work rather than be stuck in bed. Perhaps because of that, my colleagues and I did not take my condition as seriously as we otherwise would have. Finally, after nine months and more tests, my doctor found a stomach parasite. After treating it through medication, I had the energy to combat the Epstein-Barr.

Just when I felt like I was getting back on my feet, I had my second setback. In 1995, while I was cycling, a driver made a left turn directly in front of me. I slammed into the side door and sustained a minor concussion and a lower-back injury. Afterward, I could walk, but with an abnormal gait and excruciating pain. It took seventeen months of rehab, with three sessions per week of exercise, ice, ultrasound, and muscle-stimulation therapy, before I could train again.

During those months, I was continually aware of how important exercise and particularly cycling were to me. I had begun riding with some friends in 1991, and had sponsored a team so that some of them could turn pro. Four years later, the Simply Fit Cycling Team had over 200 members nationwide, including several former Olympians and a number of national and world champions. I could not imagine what my life would be like without being able to ride with them again.

Then, as luck would have it, I got a chance to develop an entire, top-flight line of sports nutrition supplements and foods. It was an opportunity to put state-of-the-art research to the test. I'm happy to tell you that not only was I competing again in ten months, but that soon thereafter, drawing from the information in this book, I won the California State Time Trial Cycling Championship.

Once I realized I could succeed as a competitive cyclist, I knew that just eating a healthful diet wasn't good enough. I needed to go beyond that and follow the guidelines that this book is based on in order to maximize my performance without getting run-down or ill. I had recommended this approach to my clients, and now it was time to take my own advice.

The next year, I trained with the national competition in mind. I ate more efficiently; and, for the first time in my life, I scheduled adequate recovery time between workouts. Not only did I win the state championship, I came in second in the Masters' Nationals. Best of all, I didn't experience any injuries, post-event depression, or fatigue.

After winning the state championship and being able to successfully make it through the nationals without illness, injuries, or post-competition burnout, I was inundated with requests from people who wanted to know the "secrets" to my improvements. This book is a result of those requests and my desire to share the research and strategy with everyone who trains or who wants to train effectively.

There's nothing magic or mysterious about the information in *Fuel Up*. Knowing what, how much, and when to eat is relevant not just for elite athletes, but for anyone who is interested in an active lifestyle. This includes weekend warriors, fitness buffs, people who want to get fit, and people who earn their living doing manual labor. The scientific research this book is based on proves that the optimal diet for performance is the same diet that most effectively promotes health and disease prevention. To my knowledge, no other diet or nutrition program makes this connection.

Why hasn't someone told you about this information before? That's a good question. In part it's because sports nutrition has only come of age in the past few years. It is recently that we learned which nutrients you need and in what amounts in the hours and, sometimes, the days, before, during, and after a workout to best promote cellular growth and repair.

That, however, is not the whole story. Many manufacturers have traditionally been more interested in selling products than in educating the public. Most of the books on the subject are geared toward health and disease, rather than performance. And, traditionally, the general public is far more interested in a quick fix or a standardized program that does everything for them.

Fuel Up does outline a program, but the guidelines are individualized for you. With a few simple calculations, you can customize the principles of sports nutrition so that your program reflects your individual nutritional requirements based upon each day's training, activity levels, or goals. It's what the luckiest professional athletes have been able to enjoy all along. Now these principles are within your reach.

That's why I am so excited about this book. As an athlete, I know the principles in it work. As a scientist and an educator, I can explain why they work. And as a nutritionist and fitness professional, I know that once you are armed with this information, you will have a much better chance of implementing the changes into your own diet and training.

PART I

RETHINKING YOUR WORKOUT

FUEL UP

U nless you're an elite athlete, you probably haven't given much thought to sports nutrition. Why would you? Until recently, even most scientists believed that the only people who needed to eat like athletes were the pro athletes, whose fates and fortunes depended upon their athletic performance.

We were wrong. In the past few years, we have learned that anyone who is active—from professional athletes to weekend warriors to fitness enthusiasts—can benefit from eating like a pro. As study after study proves, anyone who is active, works outdoors, or has a heavy manual workload will notice changes in performance, physical and emotional health, and appearance simply by eating the right amounts of the right food at the right time.

With proper nutrition and rest, you'll not only recover faster and improve your appearance or performance quicker, you'll feel better too. You won't constantly feel run-down or sore. You'll experience fewer setbacks from illness, injury, or mental fatigue. You'll be "in the zone" and be mentally and physically sharper.

To put some muscle behind these claims, I want to introduce you to four people who have benefited directly from the principles in this book. Only one of them is a professional athlete. Chances are, you'll recognize bits of yourself in each person.

Kimberly is a thirty-four-year-old who runs four or five miles a day, five times a week. She's never going to win a major race, nor would she want to. Instead, she runs to maintain her weight, stay healthy, and relieve stress. Despite this lifestyle, she was tired much of the time. She was frustrated because she wasn't getting any faster. And because she had to force herself through the workouts, they weren't as enjoyable anymore.

As it turns out, the problem had nothing to do with exercise, but with her diet. Kimberly didn't think that eating before a workout was a good idea, so she would get out of bed and hit the trail without having anything to eat or drink. As a result, she was literally running on empty.

To give her the energy she needed, I recommended that she drink a meal-replacement shake or eat an energy bar right before going out the door, and that she start carrying a water bottle on her run. She noticed a change immediately. She not only ran better, but had more energy throughout the day. The reason? She no longer had to dig herself out of the nutritionally depleted hole her morning run had created.

Nancy is in her early 70s. Reasonably active most of her life, she now goes to the gym almost every morning and does some form of weight, flexibility, or cardiovascular training. Admittedly "addicted" to exercise, she is well aware of its importance. Indeed, as her peers got sick, became hospitalized, or died, she was terrified that an injury, a fall, or worsening osteoporosis would force her to "act her age."

Because her fitness program was already well rounded, Nancy's next step was to upgrade her diet. After I analyzed it, I convinced her that she had not been eating enough protein or taking in enough fluids. Increasing her intake of protein and water, along with a calcium-magnesium-zinc supplement and a multi-vitamin, multi-mineral pill, paid off. After a recent checkup, she found that her bone loss had stabilized and her prognosis for combating osteoporosis was much improved.

Peter is an art director in his mid-40s. A father of three young children, he recently got a black belt in martial arts, routinely goes skiing, and often eats on the run so that he can squeeze in a workout. Lately, however, he hadn't been able to work through his shoulder pain, and had been taking ibuprofen three or four times a day, and in increasingly larger amounts on hard days, to "push through the pain." Knowing he had a 50–50 chance of needing shoulder surgery, he still exercised, although at a lower intensity, to maintain fitness. As hard as he tried, though, he felt like he was fighting a losing battle.

An MRI on his shoulder revealed that the injury was in the ligaments supporting his joint, not in the muscles. The first thing I did was take Peter off ibuprofen and all other over-the-counter anti-inflammatories. Rather than help, they were actually impairing his recovery process. They block pain but they also limit the connective tissue's natural rebuilding process. Thus, while masking the symptom (pain), they were hindering his body's natural healing ability. In their place, I put Peter on a glucosamine sulfate joint-complex supplement and added a more extensive stretching regimen to his training program. Six weeks later, most of his shoulder pain was gone, and Peter's doctor no longer thought that surgery was necessary.

Rob is not only a thirty-two-year-old elite athlete, but a nationally ranked triathlete who has been training for a place on the Olympic team. Although supremely gifted, he was inconsistent in his performance, and taking too long to recover, particularly on days after high-intensity interval workouts or brick workouts (in which the three sports are performed back to back). He was also constantly battling colds and upper-respiratory infections—as soon as one of his kids so much as sniffled, Rob got sick.

His problem too was primarily one of nutrition. In a mistaken belief that being as lean as possible would make him faster, he was following the Zone diet and eating meals that were relatively low in calories and composed of 40 percent carbohydrates, 30 percent protein, and 30 percent fat.

As a result, he wasn't getting enough carbohydrates or calories to perform, much less recover. I placed him on a diet geared specifically to his daily requirements. Rather than a set ratio of the energy nutrients (carbohydrates, protein, and fat), he began eating optimal levels of each and drinking more water. On some days, his ratio was closer to 70 percent carbohydrates, 20 percent protein and 10 percent fat. On other days, it was 50:30:20. I also upped his caloric intake so that he could have enough energy to compensate for the calories he burned during the workout. Each day was different because his amount of training varied from day to day.

After only several days on his new diet, he recovered faster and was performing at near-race levels with a lower working–heart rate during his workouts. In addition, his immune system dramatically improved, so that he rarely got sick.

Despite their different ability levels and athletic goals, these people are more alike than they, or, for that matter, you, might suspect. For starters, they are all athletes because they all surpass the American College of Sports Medicine (ACSM) guidelines for minimal fitness, a claim only 8 percent of the population can make.

By eating like an athlete, each of them has enjoyed a renewed sense of vitality. Kim and Peter, who were courting overuse injuries, chronic fatigue, and burnout, have nipped these problems in the bud. Rob is still closing in on his Olympic dreams; and Nancy is still in the gym, an inspiring testament to the link between fitness and longevity.

I realize this may sound too good to be true. But as our four case studies prove, unless you provide the body with adequate nutrition and fluids, workouts can actually leave you drained, sick, or injured. All four of our athletes ignored that basic fact of training. They did not replenish the nutrients they burned during exercise, and didn't give themselves time to recover properly. Once they did, they couldn't believe the difference.

If you are anything like these four, you have been trying to work through pain, make sense of a lot of conflicting information, or blindly follow someone else's recommendations. Chances are, you've never had anyone explain the basics of sports nutrition in words that you could understand. And unless you've had an expensive nutritionist or qualified personal trainer, you've almost certainly never been shown how those principles can work for you.

By the end of this book, you will have a personalized program tailored specifically to your own goals, metabolism, activity level, and taste. There will be no quick fixes, just easily digestible explanations of the program, so that you not only know how and when to eat or drink, but also why. It is that information, rather than unrealistic promises, that will give you empowering motivation to keep yourself on track.

One of the biggest differences between *Fuel Up* and most other books is that *Fuel Up* is aimed specifically at an active population. If you follow even the basic minimal standards for fitness set out by the American College of Sports Medicine, you will benefit from a more specialized, more rigorous approach to nutrition.

Because everyone's weight, metabolism, and training levels vary, the program's recommendations depend upon your weight and training intensity. Perhaps the most important difference between *Fuel Up* and most other programs is that it factors in the key variable: You.

This distinguishes *Fuel Up* from programs like the Zone or Pritikin because there is no one constant ratio of foods that you are expected to follow. These formulas, including the Zone (40% carbohydrates: 30% protein: 30% fat) and the Pritikin Foundation (75:15:10), are popular because they are simple to remember. But they don't address the fact that your nutritional needs change daily based on the amount of calories you are burning that day.

No matter how good they sound, fixed formulas aren't always realistic. As you can see by the math below, an active person on a 40:30:30 program, for instance, could be forced to eat more than 5,000 calories, 1,500 of which are from fat, a day.

Why Fixed Formulas Don't Work

Using guidelines established from scientific studies, active people need to eat 10 grams of carbohydrates and two grams of protein per kilogram (2.2 pounds) of body weight on intense training days. For simplicity's sake, let's look at the needs of a 110-pound (50 kg) female athlete and a 160-pound (72.72 kg) male athlete, each of whom has just completed a hard training day. To fully recover and benefit from the workout, they each have to eat 10 grams of carbohydrate per kilogram of body weight, or 500 grams of carbohydrate for her and 727 grams of carbohydrate for him. Since one gram of carbohydrate contains four calories, she will need 2,000 calories from carbohydrates alone.

She also has to replace protein, at the rate of two grams of protein per kilogram of body weight. That's another 100 grams of food and another 400 calories.

So far, she has put 2,400 calories into her mouth. But that's before she's figured out her daily percentage. If she were on the 40:30:30 program, she would have to eat 5,000 calories (1,500 of which are fat). That may be too high for her metabolic needs.

If she were on a restricted calorie diet, which is also in vogue again, she would have a different problem. If she were limited to 1,500 or even 1,800 calories a day, which is high for these sorts of diets, she would still be deficient not just in carbohydrate and protein, but in fat as well.

The only way she will get enough energy to recover promptly and function well is by tailoring her eating regimen so that she eats enough carbohydrates and protein to replace what she burns and to allow for full recovery. Her guidelines based on the *Fuel Up* program would be:

CARBOHYDRATE RECOMMENDATION	PROTEIN RECOMMENDATION	FAT RECOMMENDATION
(10 g / kg / day) × 50 kg =	(2 g / kg / day) × 50 kg =	67g × 9 Cal / g =
500 g × 4 Calories / g =	100 g × 4 Calories / g =	
2,000 Cal from Carbohydrates	400 Cal from Protein	603 Cal from Fat

*Nutrient recommendations and calculations are based on a 110-pound (50 kg) female, exercising vigorously and whose daily fat intake level is set at 20% of her daily total caloric intake.

Our 160-pound male athlete will require 727 grams of carbohydrate, or 2,900 calories from carbohydrate. This would be impossible to obtain on a 3,000-calorie diet or even a balanced diet of 3,500, which provides adequate amounts of protein and fat as well.

In fact, our male athlete would also require 145 grams, or 582 calories, from protein. Assuming he was taking in 10 percent of his calories from fat, he would take in 43 grams, or 387 calories, from fat for a total caloric intake of 3,877 calories to meet his nutrient requirements for this high-intensity training day. In order to obtain adequate carbohydrates on the 40:30:30 program, he would have to eat 9,667 calories!

As you can see from these examples, the nutrients that you take in daily need to be adjusted to your particular needs.

2

YOU ARE AN ATHLETE

When the importance of exercise and diet was first being trumpeted by the media 10 or 20 years ago, less than 15 percent of the country was meeting minimal levels of physical activity. Today, when the information is found in a multitude of magazines, television programs, and newspaper articles, only 12 percent are meeting that criteria.

This statistic is sobering, especially when you consider that the amount of minimal activity required is 30 minutes of physical activity every day. That's not 30 continuous minutes, mind you, but 30 minutes total, throughout the day.

It gets worse. If you evaluate people not just in terms of these minimal levels of activity necessary for maintaining health, but in terms of the minimal guidelines for fitness— essentially three 20-minute workouts at moderate intensity per week—only 7 to 8 percent of the population are active enough to reap the benefits of fitness.

That means that if you are involved in some form of regular

exercise program or sport or if your job includes a substantial amount of manual labor, you are more fit than 92 percent of the population. You may not be a threat to Michael Jordan, Venus Williams, or Lance Armstrong, but you've certainly got more in common with them than you may think.

Unless we're pros, we may feel silly calling ourselves athletes. But, according to the American College of Sports Medicine Guidelines for Fitness Training, an athlete is anyone who meets any two of these criteria:

> Participates in aerobic exercise (power walking, running, aerobic dance, rollerblading, etc.) for at least twenty minutes five times a week or sixty minutes three times a week.

> Lifts weights at least twice a week.

> Participates in yoga, dance, or flexibility exercises that utilize and stress the body on a physical level at least three days a week.

Athletic Stress

Every time you exercise, you place stress on your body. This stress, which is called exercise overload, prompts numerous physical and psychological responses called adaptations. If done properly, these responses include increased levels of fitness, strength, or power. If overdone, unchecked, or performed improperly, the responses become negative and include an increased risk of injury, a compromised immune system, and constant fatigue.

Science Matters

At any point during training, exercise alters the resting and the natural state of the body. In particular, it causes us to shift our metabolism from a phase called "anabolism" to a phase called "catabolism." Anabolism is the process of growth, repair and maintenance of cellular and bodily functions. Catabolism, on the other hand, describes the breakdown of either stored nutrients for energy or of other cellular material.

When the rate of anabolism is the same as the rate of catabolism, the body is in a state of homeostasis or maintenance. As with so many other relationships in the body, homeostasis is less a practical reality and more of a theoretical ideal. Anabolism and catabolism occur simultaneously, but they rarely occur at exactly equal rates. During exercise we're primarily in a catabolic state. Like physical trauma, exercise causes increased heat, free radical production, and cell breakage in the body. Each of these factors cause muscle damage and encourage a catabolic, or destructive, state. That continues until adequate rest and nutrients permit recovery.

Unlike other forms of stress, exercise also provides an anabolic stimulus. If the training damage is repaired with *adequate rest* and *nutrients,* exercise strengthens the muscles and other tissues of the body. At that point, the body's response shifts the metabolic and hormonal state to one that is predominantly anabolic, and therefore more conducive to growth and repair.

Stress in and of itself is neither good nor bad. On tests that rank the stress associated with life events, in fact, divorce and marriage are weighted as equally stressful. So are getting fired and getting promoted. Although one event is traumatic and the other joyous, your body's physiological responses to both type of events are the same. The actual event is less important than how you adapt or respond to it.

Thinking about exercise as a stress to the system presents a new strategy for dealing with exercise. Like all stress, it makes demands on the body—stress tears your body apart so that you can get stronger or more fit. But—as difficult as it is to believe—**you don't get fitter *while* you are working out. Your body makes the positive changes associated with the stress of the workout, such as improved cardiovascular fitness, muscle strength, tone and/or size, and increased flexibility associated with exercise in the time between workouts.**

This is a critical distinction because it explains why the recovery period is so important to your progress and health. It's not difficult in our high-achievement, results-oriented culture to see why so few people take the time to recover. The temptation to push harder and harder is reinforced by our tendency to view working through pain and "more is better" as appropriate responses. As a result, many of us actually overtrain and only become aware of the need to recover after we've pushed ourselves into an injury, an illness, or burnout. But as *Fuel Up* explains, there's no reason to wait until something goes wrong before you give your body the time and the nutrients it needs to recover from the workout.

By paying considerable attention to the nutritional and physical demands of the workout and the crucial recovery period when you are healthy, you truly are setting the stage for positive adaptations.

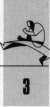

3

THE IMPORTANCE OF NUTRITION

Researchers have compared groups who eat during and after training with groups who don't. The results are always the same: Diet can dramatically improve performance and recovery.

One study by Bergstrom & Hultman, for example, measured the effect of muscle glycogen stores (carbohydrate energy stores) on athletic performance. Muscle glycogen stores directly affect how long you can maintain an activity. The subjects in the study were divided into three groups. One group ate a low (20%) carbohydrate diet; one ate a moderate (45%) carbohydrate diet; and the last, a high (70 percent) carbohydrate diet. The people in the second group whose regimen was most like the typical American diet, had half the muscle glycogen stores in their muscles than the group with a 70 percent carbohydrate diet. The second group (45 percent carbohydrate diet) could exercise only half as long, and with significantly less muscle power than the group with the higher carbohydrate intake.

Another study by Zawadzki and colleagues compared a group who ate only carbohydrates immediately after exercise with a group who ate a mixture of carbohydrates and protein, with a third group who ate placebos. The group who ate a mix of carbohydrates and protein demonstrated the most rapid and dramatic increase in muscle glycogen and recovery. While the group who ate carbohydrates alone fared significantly better than the group who ate only placebos, they were still at a disadvantage relative to the group who ate the carbohydrate-and-protein blend. This, too, is evidence of how what and when you eat affect performance and recovery.

Throughout this book, you will be reading about numerous studies that detail exactly how nutrition impacts your performance. For now, it is enough to know that nutrition is one of the most powerful weapons you have at your disposal to improve the quality of your life and the efficacy of your workouts.

Eat Like the Pros

Up until now, only a handful of professional athletes were able to make the most of their training because they had an entourage of coaches, trainers, massage therapists, and nutritionists who were paid to make sure the athlete performed at his or her best. Needless to say, most of us, including most elite athletes, don't have that sort of support. Instead, we have to squeeze our workouts in between family, work, and other activities and obligations. Because we have many demands on our time and because we don't have experts walking us through the process, we usually eat what we are used to eating, according to habits that we picked up here and there.

In addition, while there are a lot of books, celebrity infomercials, and shops promoting get-fit-quick powders or pills, most of these products are geared at an athlete wanting to get bigger, faster, stronger—tomorrow. The people who gravitate to these promises want to believe that the solution to their problem lies in one simple product. It doesn't.

The principles of sports nutrition are based upon the body's mechanism for creating energy, which provides the power to perform and adapt to physical activity. Although understanding this process is not technically necessary—you can just follow the program and guidelines—you'll be more likely to succeed if you understand the science behind the program. Knowledge is empowering: By understanding the consequences of your actions, you'll probably be more likely to think twice before doing something that interferes with your long-term goals.

As you will learn in the following sections, an effective diet provides an optimal balance of many different nutrients, all of which are necessary for optimal performance. I will cover the macro, or energy nutrients, carbohydrates, protein, and fats, which provide the energy needed for basic functions and the building blocks for growth and repair. Then I'll discuss the micronutrients—the vitamins and minerals. Although they provide no direct source of energy for the body, they are essential in small quantities because they, too, aid in metabolism, growth, and repair. And you'll find out why water is not just another critical nutrient, but possibly the most important. We would live the shortest amount of time without it, and it is the nutrient with the largest short-term impact on performance.

Great Expectations . . .

If you are already eating a relatively healthful diet, you'll only have to make minor diet and lifestyle adjustments. If you aren't, the changes will be more extensive. While you are not going to be eating donuts or a bagel with cream cheese every morning, I promise you that you will not go hungry. If, in fact, you are like most people, you will be eating more than you did before. And you'll notice dramatic improvements in how you feel and look within a month or, in some cases, days.

However good that sounds, there are limits to the improvements you will make. Unless you are a movie star or an elite or professional athlete with a full-time trainer, cook, and staff, and eight hours to train each day, you are not going to get movie-star results in two months. But if you train properly and incorporate the information about nutrition and recovery in this book, you'll achieve your personal best. That's all any athlete, professional or recreational, can ask for.

In fact, the principles of sports nutrition apply to anyone who is active, who works outside (construction workers, postal workers, or landscapers); or who lifts and carries packages all day long (delivery people or stock clerks, people in the food-service industry, mothers). If you're expending substantial physical energy, you can minimize fatigue, reduce the risk of injury, and improve your on-the-job performance by following the nutritional and hydration guidelines in this book.

And if you're active and still carrying an extra ten to fifteen pounds, you conceivably could lose six pounds of fat and add a pound or two of muscle in a month. Although you'll only lose a few pounds on the scale, you'll be thrilled by the differences in your appearance and performance.

Duration of the Program

Fuel Up is a lifelong regimen. The quantity of food you will eat will vary according to the intensity and duration of your level of physical activity. But because you want to maintain a fairly high level of fitness throughout the year, the concern for the adequate replacement of fluids, protein, carbohydrates and micronutrients that you require will be a permanent concern. Just like health and fitness.

If you really want to make the most of this program, I believe you have to be involved in the process. It is, after all, your body and your life. You are the only one who really knows how much you want to change, how hard you really work out, or how much you really eat. I will show you what and when to eat, how to train more efficiently, and even explain the science behind the recommendations. The rest is up to you.

PART II

FOOD AS FUEL

4

CARBOHYDRATES, STILL THE STAFF OF LIFE

In many ways, carbohydrates are an athlete's best friend. This group makes up the bulk of our calories because they are critical not just for energy and performance, but for recovery and repair. Despite the current—and mystifying—popularity of low-carbohydrate, high-protein diets, people who limit their carbohydrate intake not only hurt their performance and fitness levels, but often suffer lethargy and mood swings.

Carbohydrates, which are found in plant foods such as vegetables, fruits, grains, and in dairy products, take on a variety of forms. The first major division in the carbohydrate category is between simple sugars and complex carbohydrates. Complex carbohydrates are further divided into starches and fibers. Furthermore, complex carbohydrates are classified as either digestible or indigestible.

Simple carbohydrates such as those found in fruit or dairy products are called simple sugars because they are easily broken down into glucose, galactose and/or fructose, which once absorbed are converted into glucose that the body uses to fuel its cells. These sugars are rapidly absorbed and quickly enter the bloodstream. This enables their delivery to the muscles, tissues, and the brain and insures a continuous supply of energy, which those body parts need to function properly.

Do You Eat More Sugar Than You Weigh?

Monosaccharides, such as glucose, fructose, and galactose, are the simplest form of dietary carbohydrates. They exhibit varying degrees of sweetness, but all are soluble in water. This solubility allows them to easily travel through the body, and explains why they are so quickly absorbed into the bloodstream once we eat them. All monosaccharides are eventually converted into glucose in the liver, with glucose being the predominate source of energy for all cells.

Monosaccharides can be combined into disaccharides. Two molecules of glucose combine to form maltose; one glucose molecule and one fructose molecule combine to form sucrose (table sugar); one glucose molecule and one galactose combine to form lactose (milk sugar). Individuals who are lactose intolerant lack the digestive enzyme, lactase, which is necessary to completely digest and break down milk sugars. Products now exist that are supplemented with lactase to allow lactose-intolerant people to enjoy these foods.

Most foods—and all plant-based foods—have varying degrees of a variety of sugars, so sugar deficiencies are not something we have to contend with. The average American, in fact, ate 150 pounds of sucrose (table sugar) in 1995 (up 30 pounds since 1990). Because it imparts such a pleasant taste, sugars are added to virtually all processed foods during their preparation. Most of the sugar in our diets comes from these sources. Since no more than 15 percent of your carbohydrate intake should come from concentrated sugar, limit your intake of these processed foods.

Complex carbohydrates, which are called polysaccharides, take the form of digestible starches or indigestible fiber. A single starch molecule is composed of hundreds of units of glucose linked together. In the digestive tract, the molecule is broken down and absorbed as glucose. Glucose that is not immediately used is stored as glycogen in muscle and in the liver. Once your glycogen stores have been topped off, excess glucose is transported to the fat cells, converted into fat, and stored.

Fiber, the indigestible form of carbohydrate, is most often found in the plant's cell walls, and gives the plant the strength it needs to stand. Its bulk passes through our digestive tracts, intestines, and colon in a virtually solid state. Because the bacteria in these parts of the body feed off of and attach themselves to this indigestible bulk, fiber is essential to the body's elimination of waste.

There are two types of fiber. The first is water soluble, and is found primarily in fruits and oats. Insoluble fiber is found primarily in vegetables and wheat products. The insoluble fiber helps reduce the risk of certain forms of cancer (hormone-dependent tumors and colon cancer); soluble fiber decreases the risk of heart disease by lowering blood cholesterol levels. Water-soluble fiber also helps stabilize blood sugar levels, improving insulin sensitivity, and reducing the potential for fat storage.

The Simple Sugar Vs. Complex Carbohydrate Debate

We used to think that simple sugars were absorbed rapidly and lead to a rapid rise in blood glucose, while complex carbohydrates were absorbed more slowly, resulting in more stable blood glucose levels. Recent research has found that this is not true.

The indicator for how rapidly carbohydrates are digested and absorbed is called the glycemic index. In this index, foods are ranked relative to the rate of absorption and rise in blood glucose after eating pure glucose. Glucose is rated 100 so that the other foods can be easily ranked on the index.

Foods with a low to moderate glycemic index, such as pasta, oranges, and apples, are absorbed slowly, resulting in a low rise in blood glucose and correspondingly lower levels of insulin in the blood. Foods with a high glycemic index, such as potatoes, carrots, and honey, are absorbed rapidly, causing a large rise in blood glucose and blood insulin. While insulin aids in glycogen resynthesis, extreme elevations in insulin stimulate glucose and fat transport into fat cells and their storage as fat in these fat cells. This will hinder recovery and make weight loss difficult.

Rather than assuming that complex carbohydrates are the smartest choice, determine what the food's glycemic index is instead. Some simple sugars and foods containing them, such as apples and oranges, are absorbed much more slowly and result in a lower rise in blood glucose (and therefore blood insulin) than many complex carbohydrates. A person who wants to get quick bursts of energy would therefore benefit more from a potato than a banana or an apple.

GLYCEMIC INDEX OF FOODS *

LOW GLYCEMIC INDEX (LESS THAN 25)

Yogurt, low fat, artificially sweet	15	Red kidney beans	20
Peanuts	15	Cherries	23
Soy beans	18	Fructose	23
Rice bran	20	Peas, dried	23

LOW TO MODERATE GLYCEMIC INDEX (BETWEEN 25 AND 50)

Milk, chocolate, artificially sweet	25	Fish fingers	39
Barley	26	Plum	40
Grapefruit	26	Pinto beans	40
Milk, whole	28	Kellogg's All-Bran Fruit 'n Oats	40
Sausages	29	Ravioli, meat filled	41
Lentils	30	Corn hominy	42
Kidney beans	31	Mars Snickers bar	42
Black beans	31	Apple juice	42
Soy milk	31	Spaghetti	43
Apricots, dried	32	All-bran	44
Butter beans	32	Peach, fresh	44
Milk, skim	34	Mars Twix Cookie bars (caramel)	45
Lima beans, baby, frozen	34	Orange	46
Fettuccine	34	Pear, canned	46
Mars M&M's (peanut)	34	Sweet potato	46
Nutella spread (Ferrero)	34	Mars Chocolate (Dove)	46
Yogurt, low fat, fruit sugar, sweet	34	Pinto beans, canned	47
Chick peas (garbanzo beans)	34	Capellini	47
Milk, chocolate, sugar sweetened	36	Macaroni	47
Vermicelli	36	Linguine	47
Pear, fresh	39	Lactose	47
Apple	39	Cake, sponge	47
Tomato soup	39	Grapes	48
Corn tortilla	39	Pineapple juice	48
Mung beans	39	Peach, canned	49

MODERATE TO HIGH GLYCEMIC INDEX (BETWEEN 50 AND 75)

Oat bran bread	50	Muesli	58
Bulgur	50	Mango	58
Peas, green	50	Kellogg's Mini-Wheats	59
Mixed grain bread	50	PowerBar (Powerfoods)	59
Grapefruit juice	50	Pita bread, white	59
Baked beans, canned	50	Apricots, fresh	59
Chocolate	51	Honey	60
Pumpernickel	52	Bran chex	60
Ice cream, low fat	52	Rice, white	60
Tortellini, cheese	52	Rice vermicelli	60
Yam	53	Pastry	61
Orange juice	54	Kellogg's Just Right	61
Kidney beans, canned	54	Pizza, cheese	62
Bulgur bread	55	Split pea soup	62
Kellogg's Bran Buds	55	Hamburger bun	63
Kiwifruit	55	Oatmeal	63
Cake, pound	56	Ice cream	63
Kellogg's Special K	56	Muesli Bars	63
Banana	56	Mars Kudos bars (choc chip)	63
Sweet potato	56	High fructose corn syrup	65
Potato crisps	56	Apricots, canned, syrup	66
Oat bran	57	Raisins	66
Sweet corn	57	Mars Bar	66
Kellogg's Honey Smacks	57	Rye bread	67
Rice, brown	58	Semolina bread	67
Oatmeal cookies	58	Macaroni and Cheese	67
Fruit cocktail	58	Black bean soup	67
Popcorn	58	Sucrose (table sugar)	67

continued

MODERATE TO HIGH GLYCEMIC INDEX (BETWEEN 50 AND 75)

Oat bread	68	Taco shells	71
Couscous	68	Wheat bread, high fiber	71
High-fiber, rye crispbread	68	Shredded wheat	72
Cantaloupe	68	Melba toast	73
Life	69	Cream of wheat	73
Kellogg's Nutri-Grain	69	Wheat biscuits	73
Pineapple	69	Potato mashed	73
Cake, angel food	69	Life Savers	73
Gnocchi	69	Stretch-Island Fruit Leather	73
Croissant	70	Carrots	74
Grape-Nuts	70	General Mills Golden Grahams	74
Red Oval Farms Stoned Wheat Thins	70	Water crackers	74
Soft drink	71		

HIGH GLYCEMIC INDEX (ABOVE 75)

Bagel, white	75	Breakfast bar	80
Watermelon	75	Total	80
Kaiser rolls	76	Coco Pops	80
Potato, boiled, mashed	76	Cornflakes	80
Puffed wheat	76	Vanilla wafers	80
Corn chips	76	Rice cakes	80
Cheerios	77	Post Bran Flakes	83
Graham wafers	77	Jelly beans	83
Corn bran	78	Pretzels	85
French fries	78	Kellogg's Rice Krispies	85
Pumpkin	78	Potato, microwaved	85
Donut	78	General Mills Corn Chex	86
Waffles	80	Potato, instant	86

continued

HIGH GLYCEMIC INDEX (ABOVE 75)

Corn flakes	87	Glucose	100
Potato, baked	88	Glucose tablets	107
Kellogg's Crispix	90	Maltose	109
General Mills Rice Chex	93	Maltodextrin	109
Wheat bread, gluten free	94	Tofu frozen dessert, nondairy	120
French baguette	99		

*Values are from K. Foster-Powell and J. Brand Miller, *American Journal of Clinical Nutrition* (1995), and other sources.

The amount of fat and fiber in food lowers the glycemic index. Eating a food or combination of foods that include carbohydrates along with protein and fat helps to lower the glycemic index and therefore lowers both the blood glucose and blood insulin levels. A low–moderate glycemic snack during the day will help to keep blood glucose and blood insulin levels lower and your energy levels more stable. To speed recovery and enhance glycogen resynthesis, save the high-glycemic foods for immediately after exercise.

Carbohydrates and Performance

As early as 1967, Swedish researcher Jonas Bergstrom and others demonstrated the importance of carbohydrates to the quality of exercise. Bergstrom and his colleagues designed a study that looked at the effects of low-, moderate-, and high-carbohydrate diets on endurance exercise. They measured the relationship of glycogen content in the quadricep muscles to how long the subjects could maintain exercise. Their results, which have since been confirmed by many other researchers, showed that the endurance of the high-carbohydrate group was three times as great as those in the low-carbohydrate group and twice as much as the moderate-carbohydrate group.

Since those studies, we have become more aware of how important carbohydrates are to the working muscles, as well as to the central nervous system, during exercise. Under normal conditions, the brain uses blood glucose almost exclusively as its fuel. Drops in glucose levels due to short-term starvation, a diet low in carbohydrates or prolonged exercise, impair performance and brain function. Particularly during exercise, drops in blood glucose levels tied to inadequate nutrition and/or prolonged exercise can compromise brain function. Even a mild decrease in glucose levels can cause symptoms such as weakness, hunger, and dizziness and can compromise your performance and result in a loss of motivation and fatigue.

Avoiding the "Bonk"

Whether it's hitting the wall in running or avoiding the "bonk" in cycling or whatever term is used in your sport, most athletes have experienced the feelings associated with a rapid drop in blood glucose and significantly reduced liver and muscle glycogen levels. The body feels wiped out. The muscles weaken. The pace slows and sweat pours out. If ignored, the body involuntarily shakes, vision and attention span lose focus, and the skin turns pale gray in tone. Some people can continue to exercise or compete due to their extreme levels of motivation and concentration, but even these people will soon collapse from a combination of dehydration and carbohydrate depletion. Eating and drinking carbohydrates throughout long workouts or events helps prevent the bonk, delays fatigue, and gives you the energy you need to keep going.

Carbohydrates and Repair

While carbohydrates play a role in energy production, adequate carbohydrate intake also helps reduce muscle-protein breakdown. Protein serves a vital role in tissue maintenance, repair, and growth, so there will be less damage to repair.

Several studies on weight lifters have shown a quicker rate of growth and repair and less muscle-protein breakdown after exercise when the subjects took in carbohydrates and combined carbohydrate and protein supplements for up to two hours after the workout compared to subjects who took a placebo. These studies provide indirect evidence that increased post-activity amounts of carbohydrates and protein enhance recovery and adaptation. The same holds true for all athletes.

Glycogen Storage

Your muscles have the capacity to store about 15 grams of glycogen per 2.2 pounds (1 kilogram) of muscle. A 150-pound (68-kilogram) male thus can store about 1,020 grams (or about two pounds) of glycogen. If you have not provided the body with sufficient carbohydrate reserves, however, you can have much less available glycogen. Even in the best-case scenario, this glycogen is rapidly used.

The glycogen reserves are important because they are the only substance that can supply energy to the body during short term, intense exercise. As soon as the oxygen supply or body's aerobic energy pathways are incapable of meeting the muscle's needs, almost all the required energy must come from glucose in the blood or glycogen stored in the active muscle. The increased contribution of carbohydrates in intense anaerobic exercise occurs because it is the only macronutrient that can provide energy rapidly. Without it, you could not continue.

(If you are interested in the science behind energy production, refer to Appendix IV for a more complete discussion of the process.)

Regardless of the intensity, performance levels in all workouts depend upon adequate carbohydrate intake. Without it, muscle and liver glycogen are rapidly depleted. Although liver glycogen is resynthesized at a relatively rapid rate, muscle glycogen levels take at least 20 hours to be replenished after prolonged exercise. If the muscles have been severely depleted by exhaustive exercise, it can take up to 48 hours to fully restore glycogen levels. If the levels are not replaced, performance is bound to be affected, especially if you exercise daily.

Carbohydrate intake is particularly important to endurance or competitive athletes. In one study, people who exercised on successive days and ate diets composed of 40 to 60 percent carbohydrates had significantly depleted levels of muscle glycogen compared to those on a 70 to 80 percent carbohydrate diet. Other studies have shown that people on high carbohydrate diets (10 grams/kg of body weight/day) for a week maintain muscle-glycogen levels, while those on moderate-carbohydrate intake (five grams/kg of body weight/day) actually register a reduction in muscle-glycogen levels.

Carbohydrate Loading

Carbohydrates are the only macronutrient that can significantly enhance athletic performance when eaten at levels that are above those generally recommended for training and recovery. The higher the level of carbohydrates in the body prior to exercise, the longer it takes to fatigue.

For this reason, loading the muscles with glycogen prior to competition by increasing dietary carbohydrate intake in the days prior to an event is a common practice among endurance athletes. The traditional method of carbohydrate loading called for periods of low or no carbohydrates (eating less than 50 grams of carbohydrates for two to five days) followed by two days of high-carbohydrate intake. Today, athletes prefer a six-day training taper consisting of three days of moderate-carbohydrate intake (50 percent) followed by three of high carbohydrate intake (70%–75%). If the exercise overload is reduced during this period by 50 to 75 percent, muscle glycogen stores can be increased by 300 percent (from 17 grams/kilogram of body weight to 40 or even 50 grams/kilogram). Carbohydrate loading can only be performed to its maximum effect a few times a year. If done more frequently, the elevation in muscle glycogen stores is limited.

The biggest problem with carbohydrate loading is that for every gram of glycogen you store, you automatically carry an additional 2.7 grams of water. This added weight can be uncomfortable. That extra weight requires you to burn more calories during exercise and may even negate the potential benefits of the added stores. If the exercise is taking place in a hot climate, the extra water may be beneficial for temperature regulation and hydration purposes. If body weight is a factor in performance, maintain your regular diet, which should already be high in carbohydrates.

Fuel Up: Carbohydrates—The Guidelines

Rather than looking at specific nutrient needs of the athlete, many nutritionists make recommendations for nutrient intake based upon a particular ratio of the energy nutrients and a predicted level of energy expenditure. One generalized guideline for caloric intake for athletes is approximately 50 calories of food per kilogram (the equivalent of 2.2 pounds) of body weight a day. For a 150-pound (68-kilogram) person, the guidelines would be 3,400 calories. This generalized guideline once again may not provide adequate nutrients to meet the nutritional requirements for complete recovery from training.

Instead of using total calories, the *Fuel Up* program breaks these guidelines into more specific ones that are more useful to athletes. Instead of being told to get 60 to 70 percent of their daily calories from carbohydrates, a recommendation of 7 to 10 grams of carbohydrates per kilogram of body weight depending upon the athlete's training schedule is more appropriate.

Generally speaking, athletes need 10 grams of carbohydrates per kilogram of body weight on intense training days to reduce fatigue and hinder the depletion of muscle and liver glycogen stores; eight and a half grams on moderate training days and seven grams on their off, or recovery, days. On intense training days, a 150-pound (68-kilogram) athlete, for example, needs to take in 680 grams of carbohydrate (at four calories per gram), or 2,700 calories in carbohydrates alone. See Table One in the program section for complete listings of recommended daily intakes of carbohydrates based on your body weight and activity level (p. 200). For optimal replenishment, you not only have to eat enough carbohydrates, but you have to eat them at different times during the day.

During the exercise itself, you have to take in carbohydrates to maintain your strength and endurance, and drinking a sports drink containing 6 to 8 percent carbohydrates does the trick.

While water is as effective in terms of hydration, it doesn't provide the muscles with the energy they need to maintain performance. If you don't want to buy expensive sports drinks, dilute your favorite 100 percent fruit juice with an equal amount of water to obtain the optimal carbohydrate concentration. If you're going to be exercising for more than several hours, sprinkle in a little salt to account for the electrolytes you lose through sweat.

Don't wait to drink, either. Once you start your workout or race, start drinking, especially if you're training or racing in hot, humid climates. And then drink one cup every 15 to 20 minutes.

If you're one of those people who like to eat during the workout, you can get the same effect with a sports nutrition bar, gel pack, or a solid food such as a bagel, a banana, or even a sandwich, and water. This takes longer to get into your system, though, so this is an option that is better for longer endurance workouts.

To make the most of what is called the "window of opportunity," which opens one to four hours immediately after exercise, you must get adequate and proper nutrients and fluids during this time. Even if you take in adequate carbohydrates and calories later in the day, your body still won't recover from the workout by the next day. That's why you need to start consuming carbohydrates as soon as possible following exercise.

Most sports nutritionists recommend eating 50 to 100 grams of carbohydrates per hour (a bagel, two pieces of fruit, four fig bars, and most sports bars all have approximately 50 grams of carbohydrate) for the four hours after exercise. In addition, make the next meal a high carbohydrate one (150–200 grams of carbohydrate).

To further recover and adapt to the training, continue eating a balanced diet with enough carbohydrates throughout the day to meet your daily requirements. The only time you shouldn't eat carbohydrates, or any other nutrient, for that matter, is the hour before exercise. That forces the muscles to rely on stored glycogen, rather than blood glucose, for fuel, which leads to a drop in muscle performance and to premature exhaustion.

If you wake up less than an hour before you work out, eat a banana or an energy bar or drink a sports drink during your warm-up. This gives your body added nutrients and energy for your workout and allows for a more productive session because your energy stores have been depleted overnight. If you work out during your lunch hour or before dinner, you can also start with food or drink during your warm-up for additional fuel.

And remember, carbohydrates don't just work on their own. They work hand in hand with other nutrients, especially protein, for recovery and repair.

5

PROTEIN, THE ONLY MACRONUTRIENT WITH ITS OWN RDA

Protein is called the building block of life with good reason. Found primarily in foods of animal origin, such as meat, eggs, and milk, it is used in limited amounts for energy production, but its primary function is in the maintenance, repair, and synthesis of cells and tissues.

Protein enhances muscle growth, speeds the recovery process and allows the muscle to return to an anabolic state much faster. This hastens the recovery process by minimizing the normal breakdown of muscle from exercise. Consuming protein immediately after exercise (particularly in combination with carbohydrates) reduces the inflammation that normally occurs as a result of muscle damage from exercise, particularly intense workouts, and from activities with lengthening (eccentric) muscle contractions.

The National Research Council (NRC) places protein in such high regard that it has established a Recommended Dietary Allowance (RDA) for it. (Carbohydrates and fat have no such designation.) The RDA recommends 0.8 grams of protein per kilogram of body weight per day for sedentary individuals.

Most exercise physiologists and sports nutritionists feel that this amount is too low for people who are active. Active individuals require from one to two grams of protein per kg of body weight per day, assuming an adequate caloric intake. Although this is about 150–250 percent of the current RDA for protein for adults, it is in line with the standards set by the American Dietetic Association (ADA), other authoritative organizations, and the current scientific literature. While the NRC has not yet adopted a standard for active individuals, the ADA recommends a minimum of one gram of protein per kilogram of body weight, with increased requirements for infants, children, pregnant women, or during illness or exercise. More organizations will undoubtedly follow the ADA's lead.

Although protein supplies a relatively minor 5 to 15 percent of the energy during long-term exercise, it is most important in the rebuilding process after exercise. Extra protein is used to build muscle tissue and to resynthesize metabolic enzymes and other proteins involved in metabolism. To maintain the optimal environment for rebuilding, the body needs a steady supply of amino acids from protein.

Essential or Nonessential?

There are literally thousands of different kinds of proteins within your body. All are composed of chemical building blocks called amino acids. There are about 100 of these amino acids, but only 20 or so are needed to build the proteins found in the body. The body produces many of these naturally, but the other eight to ten amino acids must be obtained through your diet. These are called essential amino acids, as opposed to the ones we can manufacture naturally, which are called nonessential amino acids.

The process of protein production is complicated and beyond the scope of this book. At the risk of oversimplification, when a cell needs to build a certain protein, it assembles an assortment of amino acids that are available. It then builds the protein until it runs out of one of the amino acids. Once a single amino acid is unavailable, production of that protein stops.

To obtain the necessary amino acids, many sports nutritionists now recommend eating anywhere from one to two grams of protein per kilogram of body weight per day.

These guidelines are important because supplying the body with either too little or too much protein can cause problems. People with protein deficiencies cannot produce new tissues or protein to replace those that are lost from life's daily processes. Without adequate protein, the body cannot efficiently regulate enzyme production, function energetically, or process blood sugar or fat properly. And as with any vital nutrient, protein deficiencies can compromise the immune system, making the body more vulnerable to infection and disease.

Just as too little protein is less than ideal, too much protein can also be harmful. Excessive amounts of protein, as little as 50 percent above your daily recommendation, are associated with increased production of ammonia and urea, which are waste products that must be excreted from the body. This not only taxes the liver and the kidneys, but also increases calcium excretion in the urine and increases the risk of osteoporosis—even with an adequate daily intake of calcium.

Do You Need to Eat Meat?

Vegetarian diets became respectable in this country about 30 years ago, probably as a byproduct of the hippie lifestyle. As vegetarianism became more popular, so did several caveats associated with it. Perhaps the most widely disseminated was the belief that animal foods contained complete proteins and plant foods contained incomplete proteins, therefore, animal protein was considered to be the superior protein source. To compensate, vegetarians were given a stringent list of rules, such as eating grains and legumes in prescribed amounts simultaneously, to obtain a complete protein.

There is nothing wrong with the idea of food combining, but the process can be difficult and cumbersome to people with 21st century schedules. Fortunately, we have recently discovered that the studies we were basing our recommendations on were flawed by technical limitations and faulty hypotheses.

Researchers weren't aware that rodents, the subjects of those studies, processed protein differently than humans. Rodents, for example, have a much higher requirement for the essential amino acid, methionine, which is necessary for the growth of their fur and nails, than do humans, for obvious reasons. While it is still an essential amino acid, we need much less of it than we thought. Getting that amount from plant-based sources is not nearly the problem it was thought to be.

Additional studies based upon human needs and human subjects led to the discovery that some plant protein, particularly those based on soy sources, were as effective as animal protein. Furthermore, because isolated soy protein is devoid of saturated fat and cholesterol, it carries none of the attendant risks of cancer, osteoporosis, coronary heart disease, and early menopause that protein derived from animal sources does. Even better, it is also rich in a substance called genistein, which lowers blood cholesterol and reduces the risk of degenerative disease.

These results have spearheaded a revision of the rating system previously used to rank protein quality. The FDA used to rely on a standard called the Protein Efficiency Ratio (PER), which measured the ability of a protein to support growth in a young rat. Now it uses the Protein Digestibility Corrected Amino Acid Score (PDCAAS) for all foods intended for children over four and nonpregnant adults. Under the new, more useful banner, soy protein is ranked with milk and eggs as a perfect protein. That is welcome information not just to vegetarians, but to anyone who is interested in reducing their consumption of animal products and risk of degenerative disease.

While you can get adequate amounts of protein following a plant-based diet, it is more difficult for an athlete to obtain the higher levels needed on high-intensity training days without feeling full from the high volume of a plant-based (high-fiber) diet. Other concerns for nonmeat eating athletes include making sure they obtain adequate micronutrients such as iron and vitamin B12 and combine food sources to aid in bioavailability of micronutrients and quality protein through complementary protein sources, especially if they are vegan or are not eating soy.

The quality of protein is graded based upon the amino acid quality, quantity, and bioavailability, which is defined as the amount of a nutrient that is absorbed into the bloodstream relative to the amount ingested found in the food.

Yolk Lore

While 50 percent of the protein in an egg is in the yolk, the o⁄

white. All the fat, and cholesterol however, is contained in the ⁄

quality, the amino acid makeup of the white is comparable to the yolk. ⁄⁄⁄⁄⁄

egg whites yields as high a quality protein as eating whole eggs.

In fact, for the calorie content of one whole egg (75 calories), you can eat five egg

whites and get two and a half times the amount of protein—without the fat or cholesterol.

Egg whites either alone, in an omelet, or when used in baking (substituting two egg whites

for each whole egg in a recipe) is an excellent and inexpensive source of protein. Because

there is no fat or cholesterol in egg whites, feel free to eat them every day.

Fuel Up: Protein—The Guidelines

To get the right amount of protein for your needs, you will vary your protein intake based on your training level each day. See Table Two in the program section (p. 204) for complete listings of recommended daily intakes of protein based on your body weight and activity level. Because the amount you need is dependent upon your body weight and your exercise overload, the recommendations for protein, like those for carbohydrates, are based upon grams rather than a percentage of your overall diet.

Choose exactly how much protein to consume according to your training schedule. If, for example, you aren't training very hard, as in the off-season or when you're on vacation, your protein level is set according to the low end of the training spectrum (one gram per kilogram of body weight). During your regular training program, you will eat an additional half a gram per kilogram of body weight.

And when you're training intensively, be it for a competition or a personal goal or starting a new regimen, you'll be required to eat two grams of protein per kilogram of body weight.

Although you could conceivably consume enough protein in one sitting for the entire day, it's more effective to eat protein at every meal. Spreading it out over the course of the day helps stabilize your blood sugar and energy levels, and provides the body with a fairly steady amino acid pool to choose from. This relatively constant balance of amino acids in the bloodstream also establishes an optimal environment for growth and repair.

Protein also operates in the same window of opportunity as carbohydrates, and should be eaten during or right after a workout. Getting adequate protein into your bloodstream limits muscular and systemic catabolism because protein shifts the hormonal and cellular environment of the involved muscle into a growth mode. The quicker your blood levels of amino acids return to the pre-exercise state, the quicker cellular metabolism shifts from the breakdown of protein to synthesis of new protein.

Although less critical than carbohydrates in terms of supplying the body with energy, protein's effect on athletic performance should not be ignored. Scientific studies have shown that a group of essential amino acids, called branched-chain amino acids, behave like carbohydrates and when used during exercise reduce fatigue, prolong exercise duration and limit muscle protein breakdown.

While no specific guidelines for the amount of protein that should be consumed during the workout exist, having amino acids in your system theoretically will limit muscle protein breakdown. Recent research about protein after exercise suggests that a carbohydrate to protein ratio of anywhere from four to one to three to two significantly helps with muscle repair, and enhances the rate of muscle glycogen resynthesis. In addition to eating the recommended 50 grams of carbohydrate per hour for up to four hours after exercise, you should take in anywhere from 12 to 33 grams of protein at the same time.

Many sports bars and recovery shakes not only meet these requirements, but are more palatable immediately after a workout to many people. To make sure the product you choose is appropriate, read the label. These figures will be clearly marked.

Because your protein intake on the days of your intense workouts is twice the amount you'll be taking in on your easy days, it will seem like protein makes up the bulk of your calories. It doesn't, but it's easy to feel that way if you fill up on carbohydrates first. So that you don't deprive yourself of the necessary amount of protein, make sure you don't overdo the carbohydrates and shortchange yourself in terms of the protein.

6

"FAT," NUTRITION'S THREE-LETTER WORD

Because we are so consumed by the negative consequences of fat (largely due to media attention), we forget that fat is an essential component of our diet. To begin with, fats are the primary source of stored energy. Because they have twice as many calories as carbohydrates and protein, they contain twice as much energy per gram. If we had the capability to store an equivalent amount of energy in carbohydrates in the form of glycogen, we would weigh an additional 100 to 200 pounds.

In addition, our bodies use fat as the main source of fuel for our muscles and other body tissue while we are at rest and while we're performing light to moderate aerobic activity. They help insulate us from extreme changes in temperature and aid in the absorption of fat-soluble vitamins, such as vitamins A, D, E, and K. Also, fats add taste and texture to food.

Some Fat Is Worse Than Others

All foods contain a mixture of saturated and unsaturated fats and are classified by which type is predominant. High levels of saturated fatty acids are found in animal fat, including meat, milk, and butter. Generally, fats that come from foods of plant origin and are liquid at room temperature are either primarily monounsaturated, such as olive oil, or primarily polyunsaturated, such as corn and cottonseed oils. Fish are also high in polyunsaturated fatty acids, particularly omega-3 and omega-6 fatty acids. And certain, plant-derived "tropical" oils, such as coconut, palm, and palm kernel oil, contain a relatively high percentage of saturated fat.

Trans-fatty acids are another thing to consider. While they are not found naturally in food, they are produced synthetically when a polyunsaturated oil is hydrogenated, or has hydrogen forced into its chain. This process extends shelf life and gives the oil a semi-solid, spreadable texture, such as in margarine, salad dressing, and baked goods. Although technically not saturated fats, our body handles them as if they are.

All fats have 9 calories per gram (compared to 4 calories for carbohydrates and proteins), but saturated fats and trans-fatty acids pose particular problems to the athlete. In addition to stimulating the production of triglycerides and cholesterol in the liver, increasing the risk of heart disease, cancer, and obesity, they have a detrimental impact on performance. By changing the cell membrane properties, they decrease the cell's functional capacity and they also limit the transport and delivery of oxygen and other nutrients to the cell.

Saturated fats have been shown to increase oxidative stress on the body and limit oxygen delivery to working muscles and therefore lower aerobic capacity. Therefore, the ratio of saturated to unsaturated fat from the foods you eat is one of the most important factors in your diet. The less saturated fat you eat, the better off you'll be. A French group recently reported that masters athletes whose dietary fat contained primarily unsaturated fatty acids had better oxygenation of their blood during high-intensity exercise.

While the standard recommendation used to be to eat no more than 10 percent of your calories from saturated fat, I recommend that you get less than 7 percent of your calories from saturated fat. If you have a family history of heart disease, cancer, diabetes, or obesity, or if you have already gotten used to the taste of low-fat foods, drop the percentage and number of calories from saturated fat to 5 percent. Limiting not only total fat but the level of saturated fat to less than 5 percent of the total calories makes sense both for health and performance.

So How Much Fat Should You Eat?

While some fat is essential, too much fat is literally deadly. Excessive fat intake has been directly linked to obesity, high blood pressure, elevated cholesterol, increased risk of heart disease and cancer, and suppression of the immune system. As if that were not bad enough, unlike carbohydrates and protein, which are more easily accessed for fuel, fat in your diet is easily metabolized into stored fat. Ninety-seven percent of the excess fat you eat is directly stored as body fat.

As a result, most people need to limit, not increase, their intake of fat. There has been considerable discussion over the past 20 years regarding how much fat people should eat. Recommendations have

Science Matters

We've all heard that saturated fat is bad and unsaturated fat, particularly the monoun-saturated fats found in olive oil, is a better choice. But how many of us really know what a saturated fat is?

Between 90 to 95 percent of the fats in our diet are triglycerides, which means that they are composed of a molecule of glycerol (a three-carbon compound) combined with three fatty acids (which are primarily composed of carbon chains with hydrogen atoms attached to them). We will primarily be concerned with the three fatty acids, because they are the part of the fat that affects our performance, health, and fat-cell metabolism.

A saturated fatty acid is a chain of carbon and hydrogen atoms. Each of the carbon atoms in the chain contains no double bonds (two links holding each carbon atom together). Because there are no double bonds between carbon atoms in a saturated fat, each carbon is said to be fully saturated with hydrogen atoms. A fatty acid with one double bond is a monounsaturated fat; a fatty acid with two or more double bonds is a polyunsaturated fat.

Fats technically are solid at room temperature, oils, liquid at room temperature. The more saturated fat in the food the more solid it usually is. The tropical oils, coconut, palm, and palm kernel, are the only exceptions to this rule.

ranged from 30 percent of the diet, the standard adapted by the American Heart Association (AHA), to 10 percent, recommended by people like Nathan Pritikin and Dean Ornish. Over the past few years, many authorities have come to believe that 30 percent is too high, but that 10 percent is too restrictive.

Even though a diet with 20 percent fat is still difficult for many people to comply with, eating more than 20 percent while holding to your recommended daily total caloric intake makes it impossible to get enough of the carbohydrates and protein that you need for repair and recovery. Only ultra-endurance athletes with exceedingly high caloric expenditures can justify a diet higher in fat.

The focus of the AHA remains primarily on heart disease, weight loss, and cholesterol reduction. But to maximize athletic performance as well as to lower the risk of all degenerative diseases, 20 percent of calories from fat is superior.

Fat and Performance

Short-term performance studies and long-term epidemiological studies have found numerous negative consequences of a high-fat diet. Athletes switching from a higher carbohydrate diet to a high-fat diet experience drops in their performance. Fat decreases the body's ability to deliver oxygen to the working muscles and therefore lowers aerobic capacity. Fat also slows down the body's absorption of nutrients and thus limits the body's ability to get nutrients and fluid into the bloodstream during exercise. Furthermore, unlike carbohydrates, fat can't be used to resynthesize glucose and resupply glycogen stores.

This slowdown forces the body to rely on muscle and liver glycogen stores, which quickly get depleted, causing early fatigue. By also hindering fluid absorption, fat in turn decreases cardiovascular function and hinders temperature regulation.

Finally, most of us have too much fat stored in our bodies anyway. Depleting fat stores is not common, although some female athletes may lower their body fat levels to the point where they become amenorrheic due to a combination of factors, including inadequate energy (caloric) intake, high levels of exercise, and depressed hormone levels. Neither depleted fat stores nor inadequate dietary fat lead to this condition on their own. While a single exercise session can deplete muscle carbohydrate stores, it is not possible to deplete our body-fat stores in one workout. Given the negative impact on performance, particularly endurance performance, it is difficult to recommend a high-fat meal or, for that matter, even an exercise bar that has more than 20 percent fat.

There's Fat in Almost Everything

While we need small amounts of dietary fat for the essential fatty acids (one to two percent of total calories), there is really little need to worry about fat deficiency because virtually all foods contain fat. Even fruits, grains, and other "carbohydrate" foods, which are considered to be all carbohydrates, contain minute (and sometimes significant) amounts of fat.

For example, look at the box of oats the next time you make oatmeal. Although the only ingredient is rolled oats, a bowl of oatmeal contains three grams of fat per serving. Fat also contributes 17 percent of the total calories per serving due to the natural fat that is present in oats. Apples and other fruits contain slightly less than one gram of fat per piece. Because fat is contained in many foods, eating a diet without adding fat still provides you with all the fat you need.

Labels Are the Smart Eater's Bible

Because it is so easy to exceed the recommended amount of fat, especially saturated fat, in your diet, get used to reading labels. When you do, be aware of a loophole in the labeling laws that can make a particular food seem more healthful than it really is. As a result of a lobbying effort on the part of the food industry, trans-fatty acids are classified as part of the polyunsaturated or monounsaturated content, rather than being listed as saturated fats.

The only way to find out if a product contains trans-fatty acids is to look at the ingredient list on the label, where they will be listed as partially hydrogenated vegetable oils. So while the nutrition information will list zero saturated fat in the product if there are partially hydrogenated vegetable oils there, the truth is the fat content of the food is far more detrimental to your health and performance than you might assume.

These oils are extremely common in processed food, so your only protection is to read the ingredient list and limit or avoid products that contain them. Most sports bars that are coated with either chocolate or yogurt contain partially hydrogenated vegetable oils so read the label.

Another way manufacturers mislead the uneducated public is by labeling the fat content by percentage of weight, instead of by percent of calories. We're all familiar with the labels on dairy and meat products, which proclaim these foods to be fat-free, nonfat, or low-fat. The current labeling law for these foods allows for the content of fat to be listed based upon its percentage of weight. Because water is a principal ingredient in these foods, the percentage of fat by weight is a deceptive measurement. What you need to look for is the actual percent of calories from fat.

To see how this works, check the labels on many of the supposedly fat-free margarine and butter substitutes the next time you're in the market. A serving size of a popular fat-free, nonfat margarine for example, contains only five calories. By reading the nutritional information on the label, you'll see that while the fat grams are listed at zero grams, the calories from fat are listed correctly as five calories. Doing some simple math shows that a serving, as well as the whole product, constitutes 100 percent fat-based calories.

Manufacturers are able to list products like these as fat-free or nonfat if there is less than one gram of fat per serving. If you read the serving size on many of these products, including processed meat, fat-free candies, and snack foods or anything else that uses the term "fat-free," you may be surprised to find out how small a serving size is. You will notice that a serving of lunch meat, for example, is one thinly sliced piece of meat. If they were to label the product by a more realistic serving size, it would be more readily apparent that these foods often contain more than 50 percent of their calories in fat.

Saturated fats are now required to be listed on the label; hydrogenated fats can only be found by reading the list of ingredients. By reading the nutrient label carefully, you will find out that one small sausage link (75 percent fat calories) has 23 percent of your recommended saturated fat intake (using the excessively high 10 percent standard); and that the glass of 2% low-fat milk (37 percent fat calories) has 15 percent of the recommended daily value.

Fuel Up: Fat Guidelines

Because fat can only be used as energy or stored as fat, and because insufficient fat stores are not a problem for most of us, *Fuel Up* limits fat intake to less than 20 percent of the total calories. The total dietary fat intake will be set at either 10 or 20 percent of your total caloric intake. For weight loss, weight maintenance, or brief workouts, stay at 10 percent fat in your diet, combined with adequate protein and carbohydrate intakes. For endurance exercise, especially if it is longer than two hours, increase the percentage of fat to 20 percent of total calories. See Table Three (p. 207) for a complete list of recommendations based on body weight and activity levels.

Timing of consumption is less important with fat than carbohydrates or protein. The only times to restrict your fat intake is during and immediately after exercise, when rapid delivery of nutrients is critical and fat will slow absorption and impair the nutrients getting to the muscles quickly.

All that you have to remember with fat is to limit your intake to the percent of your calories based upon your activity level. Also be sure to stick to the prescribed five to seven percent for saturated fat intake. As much as possible avoid hydrogenated oils and trans-fatty acids.

7

DOUBLE TROUBLE—WHEN SUGAR AND FAT GET TOGETHER

I t isn't only the general population that has weight-loss concerns. Athletes in a wide variety of sports are concerned not only with appearance, but the effects of extra body weight on performance. While there have been hundreds of diets to come out that work for the short term, that weight loss usually doesn't last. Not only that, while losing weight on those diets, you generally feel sluggish and weak—qualities not consistent with those most athletes, if not most people, desire.

Caloric Balance

Most people don't really understand the roles exercise and diet play in weight loss, particularly their effects on metabolism. It all comes down to the concept of caloric balance.

Caloric balance is a function of caloric intake, or the amount of calories you eat each day, and caloric expenditure, which is the number of calories you burn. If you eat more calories than you burn, these calories are stored as fat. If you burn more, you have a caloric deficit. If you've done it right, with a program of balanced nutrition and regular exercise, you'll be able to access stored calories and lose weight. Fortunately, both caloric intake and caloric expenditure are factors that we can modify and control.

To understand exactly how the two interact, consider examples from both extremes of the spectrum. At one end are the ultra-endurance athletes. Although they can eat 8,000 to 12,000 calories a day, they only have 4 to 6 percent body fat. That is because they exercise for six to eight hours a day, and have trained their metabolisms to be incredibly efficient at converting food to useable fuel, rather than fat.

At the other end of the spectrum are overweight people with excess body fat who regularly ingest only 2,000 or even 1,000 calories a day. They have such sluggish metabolisms that even the sparse amount they eat is stored, rather than burned, leaving them with body-fat levels of 20 to 30 percent or more. Their experience proves that body composition isn't as much a question of how many calories you eat as of how many you burn.

In theory, at least, losing weight is simple: Burn more calories than you eat. Because a pound of body fat contains 3,500 calories, you lose a pound of weight each time you use 3,500 calories more than you take in.

There are three ways to develop this kind of caloric deficit. First, you can eat less. Secondly, you can eat the same, but increase the number of calories you expend by exercising. Third, you can eat less and work out more.

In the short run, it doesn't matter which option you choose. The long run, however, is entirely different. Reducing your caloric intake by anything over 250 to 300 calories a day is an invitation to failure. When you eat less, your metabolism's efficiency drops anywhere from 7 to 80 percent. On average, people will experience a 20 percent decrease in metabolic efficiency. This slowdown makes it very easy to regain the weight.

Because exercise, and resistance training in particular, raises the metabolic rate, you can lose weight simply by upping your exercise level. But 3,500 calories is a lot to shave off by workouts alone. As a result, it is probably easiest to lose weight by cutting out 250 calories a day (one candy bar, half a donut, a handful of chips) and exercising regularly. That way, you can lose one to two pounds a week (or, if you're over 200 pounds, 1 percent of your body weight).

That might not sound dramatic, but it is the safest, most effective amount to lose. If you lose more weight faster, you'll be losing water and lean body weight, which in turn undermines your ultimate goal of improving your body composition. Moreover, because this slower weight loss is associated with an improved metabolism, it tends to be weight that stays off.

The Mechanics of Fat-Cell Metabolism

Because of genetics and personal history, some people will have an easier time losing weight than others. That inequality can usually be traced to when and how they put on the excess weight in the first place. Because this difference can be frustrating, the awareness of these factors is critical to the establishment of realistic goals.

Overweight people generally fall into one of three categories. In the first, a condition called hyperplasty, or hyperplastic obesity, the person has more fat cells than average. In the second, hypertrophy, or hypertropic obesity, the size of the fat cells are larger than average. In the third, hyperplastic-hypertropic obesity, the person's fat cells are both larger and more numerous than average. Many of these individuals who have gained weight their entire lives are considered morbidly obese. (This means that more than 50 percent of their body weight is body fat. Because their situation is more complicated, the morbidly obese should undergo weight-loss programs in conjunction with a qualified physician or health-care professional.)

At this point in your life, you can't do anything about the number of fat cells in your body. A normal individual has about 25 billion of these cells. This number can be increased during infancy, puberty, and with excess weight gain (generally greater than 40 pounds) during pregnancy. It can also be increased during the period of rapid weight gain that follows temporary weight loss throughout your life. These added fat cells are the real danger to caloric reduction and to weight cycling.

Typically, hyperplastic individuals were heavy as children or adolescents, and have been battling weight problems all their lives. Hypertropic people typically were lean through their teen years, but have put on a few pounds a year ever since. By the time they hit their late 30s, they are about 20 pounds heavier than they should be.

This kind of weight gain is called "creeping obesity" because the weight was put on gradually, after puberty. Rather than a result of additional numbers of fat cells, it is marked by a swelling of the existing fat cells. In most cases, the cells are 30 to 40 percent larger than they were when the individual was lean.

Although hyperplastic people may find weight loss slightly more difficult than hypertrophic individuals do, the difference between the two is most readily apparent during the weight-maintenance phase of the weight-management program. A hypertrophic individual only has to shrink the fat cells back to their original size. Once that happens, his or her metabolism returns to levels that are only about 100 calories a day slower than it was in their early 20s. Since the hyperplastic individual still has the same number of fat cells he or she did when they started the diet, their metabolisms will be less efficient. Although they too can still stay relatively lean, they have to remain more vigilant. They may also have to accept being slightly heavier than they would like. The few extra pounds pose no health risk or insurmountable threats to their self-image or appearance.

Turn Up the Heat

Changing your fat-cell metabolism involves two separate processes: the rate at which fat is stored, and the rate at which it is removed from fat stores. Each process requires a different enzyme. Lipoprotein lipase (LPL) affects fat storage; hormone-sensitive lipase (HSL), affects the removal of fat from a cell.

Think of these two enzymes as if they were light bulbs on a dimmer switch. When the LPL is stimulated, or when its switch is on high, the body stores fat. When it is less bright, or less active, and the HSL's switch is intensified, the body is more likely to release the stored fat. Numerous stimuli exist for each of these enzymes, many of which are present at all times, at various levels. Our body's decision to either store or remove fat is a result of the interplay of the stimuli on these enzymes, which are always active, but operate at varying levels of activity.

Fat Storage

Each enzyme has its own set of stimuli. LPL is attached to the membrane outside the fat cell. As soon as you eat something, you increase the amount of fat or insulin (primarily as a result of blood glucose changes) in the bloodstream. These changes cause the LPL to be more active. This in turn alerts the fat cells. By the time the fat reaches the cell, these cells are ready and waiting to store it.

To derail the fat-storage system, you have to limit the amount of fat and concentrated sugars that you eat. Doing so triggers other favorable hormonal changes, such as the lowering of insulin levels in the blood. Because insulin is the second primary controllable activator of LPL, a limited intake of fat and concentrated sugars is doubly important and doubly effective.

Besides the amount of particular nutrients, overall caloric intake also affects LPL. Severe caloric restriction (a caloric deficit of more than 300 calories a day), results in an increase of LPL activity. Because your body is burning more calories than you have taken in you not only lose weight during the caloric restriction, but also the size of your fat cells decrease. However, as the cells decrease in size the number and activity of LPL enzymes on each fat cell increases. Although it is possible to lose weight on diets designed around severe caloric restriction, the increase in LPL activity sets us up for weight regain upon resumption of our old eating patterns. In fact, 95 percent of those who lose weight regain it within two to five years.

Fat Removal

If a good diet is the key to reducing fat storage, regular exercise is the secret to fat removal. HSL is activated not by food, but by the increased production of a hormone called epinephrine, which itself is stimulated by exercise. This increased activity in HSL remains elevated as a result of exercise training.

An additional beneficial hormonal adaptation resulting from exercise is the body's improved ability to regulate blood sugar by lowering insulin levels in your bloodstream at all times, including after meals. That helps tell the body to burn, rather than store, fat.

Insulin is one of the primary stimulants of LPL. Both diet and exercise play a key role in regulating your blood insulin levels. Foods that are highly concentrated with sugar stimulate insulin release and therefore stimulate fat storage. Many of the supposedly healthful fat-free products are calorically dense due to high amounts of added sugar. While they may technically be fat free, they definitely encourage fat storage.

Exercise also helps counter the effect of excess calories derived from carbohydrate and protein sources. If you eat too much of these foods yet exercise regularly, the body burns up not just what it needs for the exercise, but much of the additional carbohydrates and proteins circulating in the bloodstream as well.

Excess fat, however, is not subject to this safeguard. While excess carbohydrates and protein can virtually burn themselves up with exercise, dietary fat does not readily make itself a fat-burning fuel. That is why almost all of it ends up in the fat cells.

Through dietary and exercise changes (including limiting fat intake and an increase in daily activity), it is possible to reestablish a metabolism that is efficient at removing and burning fat and inefficient at storing it. You can see that it's important to maintain an adequate caloric intake by eating all your meals as well as snacks daily. By eating throughout the day, you're helping to maintain an environment that leads to weight loss, recovery, performance, and optimal health.

Keep in mind that while we have no control over some of the factors that affect LPL and HSL, others can be modified through diet and exercise, both of which we do have control over.

Exercise

Exercise is the next big piece of the puzzle. Despite the media's ongoing blitz on fitness, America is fatter and more unfit than ever. Fewer than 8 percent of the population get enough exercise to comply with basic fitness guidelines. And the situation gets worse each year.

One of a host of problems associated with the lack of exercise is its effect on long-term weight loss. A definitive study of two groups of people in weight-loss programs proves why. One group in the study lost weight by cutting calories; the other group lost weight by changing their eating habits and exercising regularly.

Both groups lost the same amount of weight, which was expected since they took in and expended the same number of calories. But the group who cut calories lost half the weight from their body-fat stores and half from lean body mass, while the group who exercised lost no weight from their lean body mass. Instead, all the weight they lost came from their body fat. Although the participants weighed the same, the second group had altered their body composition so that they could keep the weight off. The group who had merely dieted, however, were positioned to regain the weight.

The important lesson in this study is that exercise improves your body composition, or the percentage of body fat to lean muscle mass. Because exercise burns fat and builds lean muscle tissue, it not only causes you to lose weight, but also gives you less body fat relative to the amount of lean muscle mass in your body. Because one pound of lean muscle requires as much as ten times as many calories at rest as a pound of fat, you can eat more calories than you otherwise would before gaining weight. If, as the result of training you gain one pound of muscle and lose one pound of fat, your caloric requirements will increase by 35 calories per day. Replacing four pounds of body fat with four pounds of muscle, which is realistic under any balanced weight loss and exercise program, will increase your caloric requirements by 140 calories per day, almost 1,000 calories a week.

Building Muscle Burns Fat, Even When You Sleep!!

Traditionally, aerobic exercise is associated with weight loss. When one thinks of weight lifting, the first vision that comes to mind is of a highly muscled, rather than a lean, athletic physique. But while cardiovascular exercise is a principle component of any exercise program for weight control, resistance (weight) training appears to be vital in order to maintain and/or increase lean muscle mass—a necessary component for increased metabolism and weight maintenance.

For most individuals, the basal metabolic rate (BMR), or the amount of calories necessary to maintain the body at rest, comprises the greatest component of their daily energy expenditure. The amount of lean body (muscle) mass an individual has is a prime determinant of their BMR.

BMR can be measured in a medical laboratory or can be estimated by multiplying your body weight in pounds by 10 if you are a woman, and 11 if you are a man. This value is modified based on numerous factors including the type of diet you are on, your activity level, your body composition, your health status, and your genetics. Since you have control over some of these factors, the final figure is not as simple as straight multiplication.

BMR does not take into account the energy expenditure of daily and athletic activities. For most individuals, the BMR makes up over 70 percent of their overall daily energy expenditure. The rest comes primarily from daily activities and sports and recreation. Generally speaking, at any given weight, the higher your BMR, the less body fat you will have. Exercise not only helps burn unwanted fat, but alters your body composition toward one that helps your metabolism burn fat more efficiently.

As mentioned earlier, body weight is determined by how many calories you are storing, and therefore is dependent on a balance between caloric intake and caloric expenditure. When you eat more than you expend, you gain weight and add to your fat stores. When you eat less than you are expending, you lose weight because you remove fat from those stores. By incorporating a resistance training program to your overall exercise program, you help to permanently shift your expenditure component of the equation and reduce the amount of stored fuels, primarily fat.

Some calories are expended during resistance-training workouts, but they are minimal when compared to the amount expended in a similar length aerobic workout because the resistance workout is intermittent rather than continuous. The on-time (amount of actual working time) is significantly less during a resistance workout. However, the increase in lean body mass helps to elevate the metabolism 24 hours a day, making for a significant increase in caloric expenditure over days, weeks, and months. The ACSM, therefore, now recommends two sessions of resistance training per week along with three to five sessions of aerobic exercise for adults interested in developing and maintaining cardiovascular fitness, body composition, and muscular strength and endurance.

This cardiovascular exercise should use large muscle groups, be maintained continuously, and be rhythmic and aerobic in nature, such as walking, hiking, running, jogging, bicycling, cross-country skiing, rowing, stair climbing, skating, swimming, and various endurance game activities. The ACSM recommends participating in these activities three to five days per week for 20 to 60 minutes of continuous activity at an intensity of 65 to 90 percent of your maximal heart rate. (The procedure for measuring your maximal heart rate is detailed in Chapter 10, pg. 115.) This range is defined as the person's target heart rate or training sensitive zone.

If you are interested in weight loss, as opposed to weight maintenance, longer, more frequent workouts are preferable. Varying the intensity from day to day with hard workouts separated by at least one day of an easy workout will allow you to recover and maintain your exercise frequency.

How Many Calories Do You Need to Burn?

If you are trying to burn fat and lose weight, you are going to have to spend at least 20 minutes three days per week at exercise intensities sufficient to burn approximately 300 calories. If you can't do that, you must burn at least 200 calories four times per week. This is the minimum. Programs of less participation generally show little or no changes in body composition. If the primary purpose of an aerobic workout is for weight loss, regimens of greater frequency and duration of training and moderate intensity are recommended.

If you are interested in losing weight, a one- to two-pounds-a-week weight loss from body fat stores is safest and most realistic. Losing more weight from fat is physiologically impossible. If you lose more weight than that, as some diets suggest, it's not coming from fat, but from loss of water and muscle tissue.

This is particularly important to athletes, who can't afford to simply lose weight because performance is so directly related to muscle power. Repeated studies have shown that weight loss through caloric restriction results in a significant loss of muscle (often up to 50 percent of the weight loss).

To reach a weekly 3,500 caloric deficit (one pound of body fat), you should cut 250 calories a day out of your diet. That gets you to 1,750 calories. The other half must come from exercise.

Once you know how many days a week you can work out, divide the number of days into 1,750. That will give you the number of calories you have to burn during each session. Generally speaking, moderate intensity cardiovascular workouts burn about 350 calories in 45 minutes.

If you're interested in weight loss, limit your total fat intake to less than 10 percent of your total calories. (To determine your recommended amount, use the 10 percent level for fat in Table Three (p. 207). In addition, you'll want to eat less calories in general, which also means you are going to have to reduce the amount of carbohydrates you take in. The amount will vary from day to day based on your activity level, so you'll have to use Table One (page 200) to determine your specific total daily carbohydrate requirements. On your easy, or off-days, reduce your level of carbohydrate intake to 5 grams per kilogram of body weight per day. The reduction from 20 percent to 10 percent in fat intake and the modest reduction in carbohydrates will result in the 250-calorie deficit necessary for weight loss.

The timing of weight loss is also critical for the athlete. Because energy levels for recovery are compromised by reduced carbohydrate and caloric intakes, losing weight in the off-season or early part of the season will avoid drops in energy, which is imperative for competition. Moderate caloric restriction also complements the high volume, low intensity nature of training during preseason training.

For those beginning an exercise program for weight loss, consult your physician and progress gradually. This is especially important for individuals with a history of the following risk factors for coronary heart disease: diabetes, hypertension, high blood cholesterol levels, family history of heart disease, cigarette smoking, or obesity.

If you miss a workout, don't cut back on calories to compensate for it. If you do, your metabolism will start to slow down. Console yourself with the reminder that exercise is a stress, and that your body uses recovery time to adapt to that stress. Even on a down day, you still need proper nutrition so that your body can recoup from the workout. Rest, sufficient calories, and the right nutrient balance are all essential to the process. Sometimes skipping a workout can be more beneficial than pushing past your limit.

Appetite

As you know from personal experience, you eat for any number of reasons. These cues can be divided into two basic types: the internal, or physiologic messages, and the external, or environmental ones.

The overriding internal cue to eat is hunger, which is our innate drive to eat as many calories as we need to maintain our caloric expenditure. Scientists believe that hunger is stimulated by an assortment of internal cues, including the type and amount of food in your stomach and small intestine, levels of various chemicals in the blood, and signals in the brain stimulated by amino acids, hormones, and neurotransmitters.

There is also evidence that the liver affects appetite by helping to regulate levels of circulating nutrients, such as fat, glucose, and amino acids; hormones, such as insulin and serotonin; and other chemicals. Then the nervous system integrates these messages and interprets them as "hungry" or "full." One of the roles of the liver, and in particular liver glycogen stores, is to regulate blood sugar levels. Between meals, as blood sugar levels drop due to the removal of glucose from the blood into the working tissues, the liver breaks down glycogen to supply the blood with glucose. This drop in blood sugar is one of the stimuli for hunger.

Because dietary fructose goes preferentially to the liver to resupply and help maintain liver glycogen stores, eating fruit and other foods containing fructose will help to resupply liver glycogen and suppress the appetite. Two side effects of an excessive intake of fructose, however, are gastrointestinal distress and elevated blood triglyceride levels in some individuals who have a family history of heart disease.

Aside from the chemical stimuli, we also eat when we're not really hungry. We often eat too much food if we love the taste; or get "talked into" eating just because we happen to have food placed in front of us. We eat at parties and at meetings, we eat when we're happy, we eat when we're sad, and we eat when we're bored. These are psychological, emotional, and social triggers to our appetite and are every bit as powerful as their internal counterparts.

These cues cannot be dismissed. Regardless of why you are eating, hunger is a powerful biological drive. Because it cannot be resisted over time, it is very important that anyone interested in weight loss and weight management do everything in their power to understand how these external cues manipulate their behavior. It is equally important to eat a diet that is designed to maintain blood nutrient levels, rather than cause the nutrient levels to swing from one extreme to the other.

A Special Case: Gaining Weight

Many athletes are interested in changing their body composition. Those interested in weight loss can expect to lose one to two pounds a week on a balanced weight-loss program, which combines a daily 250 calorie reduction in food and an expenditure of 250 to 750 calories in exercise, above your normal level.

This poses a problem for the athlete who is interested in gaining weight. Gaining weight per se is often relatively easy and an enjoyable task elicited by shifting the body's energy balance to a greater caloric intake. While an excess intake of 3,500 calories results in a body-weight gain of about one pound in a sedentary individual, the excess is stored as body fat.

No athlete wants this. Instead, they want to increase their body weight in the form of lean tissue, and, more specifically muscle mass. Generally, this form of weight gain is only accomplished if an increased caloric intake accompanies an appropriate exercise program. Although endurance exercise can increase fat-free body mass slightly, the body composition change is frequently accompanied by a loss in body weight resulting from fat loss. This drop in body weight is the result of the calories burned and the appetite-supressing nature of endurance exercise.

A more successful option is heavy resistance training. When accompanied with a balanced diet, it will effectively increase muscle mass and strength. To gain a pound a week of lean tissue, 700 to 1,000 additional calories per day are recommended. In addition, slightly increase your protein intake by five to ten grams per day with the remaining calories coming from carbohydrate sources.

Just as it's possible to only lose one to two pounds a week of body fat, it is also possible to only gain one to two pounds per week of lean tissue. Obviously those further from their genetic limits (the beginner) can expect this level of increase. Athletes who have relatively high testosterone levels and greater percentages of fast-twitch muscle fibers increase lean tissue to the greatest extent. One way to verify whether the combination of a higher caloric intake and heavy resistance training increases lean muscle tissue and not body fat is to regularly (weekly or biweekly) monitor your body composition at your doctor's office, local gym, or health club, rather than changes in your body weight as registered by the bathroom scale.

Eight for Ate: Helpful Hints to Keep You on Track

1. By training regularly, your overall caloric intake will be higher than when you were sedentary or not training as intensely. Consistent training will allow you to cut yourself some slack when it comes to dietary transgressions. Training gives you a little more leeway both in terms of quantity and quality of favorite foods you can enjoy—occasionally.

2. Often your appetite is reduced right after a workout and you won't feel like eating. But remember the important "window of opportunity" for muscle glycogen resynthesis. If you restore your liver glycogen stores shortly after exercise, you will be less likely to feel famished later in the day, which leads to overeating. Aside from getting carbs in, taking them partly in the form of fruit or fruit juice will supply your body with fructose, which goes preferentially to the liver and aids in restoring the liver's glycogen stores for later use. This will prevent those drops in blood glucose later in the day and ward off those serious hunger pangs that lead to uncontrolled eating.

3. Turn off the television. While the physiological mechanism remains unknown, your metabolic rate watching television is 7 to 14 percent lower than it would be if you were sitting doing nothing at all. To make matters worse, while you watch, you are bombarded by a steady stream of ads for fatty foods. If you normally watch three hours a day, which is well below the national norm, you would save 300 calories a week simply by turning off the TV. If it means you'll snack less, you could save thousands more.

4. When you're eating out, assume the worst. While much has been made about the low-fat options available in fast-food restaurants, these places are temples of temptation. We don't send alcoholics into bars, so there's little reason why you should subject yourself to a test of willpower. Are you really going to be able to order a baked potato without the butter or the sour cream? Even if you do, there are few truly nutritious items on the menu. The lean meats, when you can find them, still contain at least 50 percent fat. The low-fat shakes are mostly sugar. And the salads are usually prepackaged, tasteless, and less than satisfying. While you sometimes have no choice but to patronize fast-food outlets, do so sparingly.

5. Although many of your family and friends will congratulate you on your decision to train and compete or to lose weight, you will soon notice that some of these people, consciously or unconsciously, are not acting in your best interests. The sabotage may be in the form of little verbal digs, requests to skip a workout, or tempting you with your favorite desserts.

Their reasons for wanting you to fail can range from their concern that you won't need them once you are thin or in shape, to thinking you aren't as much fun anymore. In any case, they put you in a dilemma. If you deal with it directly, you or they are likely to get defensive. If you let it go, you may feel compromised or uncommitted.

The best advice for dealing with these diet saboteurs is to stay centered and loving. Follow your heart, and learn more about yourself and them in the process. Above all, remember that they probably are feeling attacked, threatened, or victimized by your new determination. After all, they have more important things to worry about than whether you ate a potato chip or a carrot. Over time, they will come to terms with the changes you have made. Indeed, if you don't pressure them but lead by example, they may even decide to make changes of their own.

6. Because eating is one of life's great pleasures, many of our social and professional activities revolve around food. Rather than feel like you have to eliminate your favorites and deny yourself, limit your indulgences to small, yet manageable portions. To control your urges, get in the habit of putting half a meal in a doggie bag right away and then giving it to a homeless person, sharing the food with a friend during the meal, or even throwing it out immediately, while your resolve is still strong.

7. No food is forbidden. As long as you eat it infrequently, the nutrients won't have a noticeable effect on your health and performance. Make sure to enjoy it. Don't eat it in the car or when you are reading a newspaper. And don't feel the need to eat it behind closed doors. There's nothing embarrassing about eating anything, especially if you're in control.

8. Work on your self-esteem. When you achieve a goal, celebrate. If you come up short, ask yourself if the goal was unrealistic or what you could have done differently to achieve it. Rather than focus on it as a failure, remind yourself that you are still better off than when you began the program. Then remind yourself that difficulties, struggles, and mistakes are opportunities to learn and grow.

8

(DE)HYDRATION

Water, Water Everywhere

Nutrition is not just a matter of eating right, but of drinking enough of the right kinds of fluids. In fact, you will die of dehydration well before you die of starvation. I cannot overemphasize the importance of hydration. Drinking enough water prevents both mental and physical fatigue, and is essential to effective waste removal, appetite control, and overall metabolism. And it's particularly important with regard to exercise.

As little as a 2 percent drop in hydration—which happens well before you notice being thirsty—results in a 10 percent decrease in performance. A 5 percent drop results in a 30 percent drop in performance. These drops in performance are not limited to the athletic arena. Being poorly hydrated may help explain why you feel sluggish, bored, and irritable in the afternoon. If you are at all typical, you may be in a state of partial dehydration from drinking coffee and diet soda all morning rather than water, milk, or juice.

Fortunately, few areas of sports nutrition research in recent years have been studied as extensively as that regarding fluid intake and exercise. As studies have confirmed, drinking during the workout or event negates many of the problems of dehydration on cardiovascular function and temperature regulation. We also know how performance can be improved by adding carbohydrates to the rehydration solution, and how drinking after exercise is one of the best ways to enhance and facilitate recovery.

Water and Performance

To prevent dehydration, many authorities recommend drinking a minimum of eight to ten 8-ounce glasses of water per day. For individuals engaged in exercise, both the ACSM and the National Athletic Trainers' Association (NATA) have established additional hydration guidelines.

Eight glasses of water might not seem like a lot, but most of us still don't meet these basic hydration guidelines. This may be because thirst is an unreliable indicator of fluid needs and because many people ingest excessive amounts of liquids containing diuretic agents, including caffeine, alcohol, artificial sweeteners, megadoses of water-soluble vitamins, and certain drugs, which increase urine production and dehydration.

Coffee, diet sodas, beer, other alcoholic drinks and, surprisingly, many sports energy drinks and gel packs, which contain caffeine or other stimulants such as ma huang and gurana, all contain these products. These diuretic agents compound the dehydration associated with exercise. To compensate for the effects of these caffeinated beverages or diuretic agents, you have to drink twice their volume in water in addition to your normal requirements.

Exercising in Hot Weather

The decreases in performance due to dehydration are even more severe when you work out in hot or humid weather. Not only do you sweat more, but the humidity also limits, sometimes severely, evaporative cooling. Because sweat doesn't evaporate and sits on your skin, the heat cannot be released.

That is why 100-degree heat in a dry environment like Palm Springs, California, seems cooler than an 80-degree day with 90 percent humidity in Orlando, Florida. The tropical air is already saturated, so the sweat cannot evaporate and rolls off of your body, preventing thermoregulation.

This problem is compounded by inadequate fluid intake because dehydration limits your ability to sweat and dissipate heat efficiently. The effects can be shocking. During prolonged exercise in the heat, you can lose one to two liters of fluid and two to four pounds of body weight per hour. Each pound corresponds to 16 fluid ounces (475 ml) of water and electrolytes. This loss can elevate the heart rate, decrease cardiac output, and raise the body's core temperature.

If you are interested in performing well and staying healthy, you have no choice but to replace these fluids by drinking water and sports drinks before, during, and after the workout. That is the only way you'll replenish the nutrients you lose.

The Importance of Gastric Emptying

Hydration is not just a matter of how much you drink, but of how much you absorb. The absorption of fluid and nutrients is greatly affected by several factors, including temperature, volume, carbohydrate content, and exercise intensity. Although it is often difficult to keep fluids cold during exercise, the colder the fluid you drink, the faster it will be absorbed. The more you drink at one time, the better as well. It's not always easy to rehydrate during exercise because you can often take in only a few sips at one time. Drinking more can interfere with your breathing, so this may be something you'll have to get used to over time.

Rehydration drinks with 6 to 8 percent carbohydrates are absorbed as fast or faster than water. Soda, juices, and recovery drinks, on the other hand, typically contain 12 to 14 percent carbohydrates, which limits the body's ability to absorb them during exercise.

The final factor affecting fluid absorption is exercise intensity. As long as you aren't anaerobic, the intensity of your exercise should not affect your ability to absorb fluids. If you are anaerobic, slow your pace slightly before you drink. If you are doing an anaerobic exercise, such as weight lifting or tennis, only drink between sets.

Can You Drink Too Much?

Although most of us don't drink enough, some athletes have actually died by drinking too much. Several ultraendurance athletes and marathon runners have died in the past few years, including a

The Funnel Effect

When you're in a race, remember to take a drink at every aid station along the way. And don't just take a gulp and throw the cup away. Push together the top sides of the cup to create a funnel and sip the liquid until it is all gone. There's no need to drop your cup within feet of the feed zone. Also, remember to practice drinking while you train to get your body accustomed to taking in fluids (and solids) during exercise. You eventually will be able to do it without discomfort.

woman who ran the Houston Marathon in April 2000, by drinking excessive amounts of water to compensate for fluid loss. Other athletes have experienced symptoms ranging from fluid accumulation in the lungs, brain swelling, respiratory distress, coughing, low blood-oxygen levels, frequent urination, and low blood sodium.

The condition is called hyponatremia or, in lay terms, water intoxication. Although it is relatively uncommon and should not be used by most people as an excuse to drink less, it is something to be aware of, especially in hot climates. It occurs when athletes who sweat profusely drink water or juice rather than an electrolyte recovery solution that restores blood sodium levels to normal.

Athletes who are in endurance events that last for four hours or more are at most risk, but anyone who sweats in a hot environment for hours on end must balance their sodium and water intake. In these instances, sports drinks or lightly salted water or fruit juice or a vegetable juice, such as V-8, which already has sodium, are the only liquids that work. You could also include salty food in your diet on the days when your workouts or events last for more than four hours.

Medical attention is essential if your condition becomes serious.

As was the case with several Houston Marathon runners who survived, treatment can include the use of intravenous fluids containing large amounts of sodium.

The Hydration Guidelines

To prepare for exercise and the other demands of the day, you must drink eight to ten 8-ounce cups of water a day. In addition, you should drink two to three cups of fluid two hours before you work out, and one to two cups 15 minutes immediately before the exercise. It is best to drink only water in the hour before the workout.

If you have access to a scale, weigh in, without your clothing if possible, before and after exercise. Then over the next several hours after the activity, drink two cups for each pound of weight you lost, making sure that by day's end, your body weight has returned to its preexercise level.

Although it doesn't have to be hot or humid to dehydrate yourself, it is possible to drink enough during the workout to not lose fluids. But even if you pay strict attention to your body's hydration needs, you cannot keep up with the loss while exercising in a hot environment during exercise. You will have to make up for it afterward.

For exercise shorter than 90 minutes, the ACSM recommends drinking at least one cup of fluid every 15 to 20 minutes. For longer periods of activity, you'll need a rehydration beverage containing carbohydrates in a 6 to 8 percent solution and electrolytes, to help replace those that are lost during the activity. A 150-pound person can meet his/her carbohydrate and fluid recommendations during

Yellow Is the Color

One way to tell if you are adequately hydrated after exercise is to pay attention to the color of your urine. If it is bright yellow in color, then in all likelihood, you are still partially dehydrated. Continue to drink fluids until your urine becomes faint yellow in color.

Although the frequency of urination and the color of your urine is a good indicator of your hydration levels, other factors can contribute to the color of your urine. Taking large amounts of the water soluble vitamins, particularly vitamin C, will make your urine brighter in color, as will several phytonutrients including the aspragine and aspartic acid found in asparagus. Generally your urine will have a greenish tint and slight odor due to the presence of aspartic acid after a meal containing asparagus.

prolonged exercise by drinking 625–1,250 ml (16 to 32 ounces) of beverages containing 6 to 8 percent carbohydrate per hour of exercise.

Of the numerous varieties of sports drinks on the market, the ones labeled sports hydration drinks, as opposed to recovery drinks, are formulated to conform to this range of carbohydrates. Fruit juices range between 10 and 12 percent and can be diluted one to one with water to meet the optimal concentration for fluid absorption. To improve absorption, sprinkle some salt into the juice.

Some sports drinks contain caffeine and/or carbonation. While the caffeine-laced drinks are advertised as energy boosters, they act as diuretics. Despite improving performance, they dehydrate you and are thus ill-advised choices for rehydration. Carbonation neither hinders nor enhances hydration, so carbonation is strictly a matter of taste.

Although the ACSM guidelines for workouts that last less than 90 minutes dictate drinking water rather than sports nutrition drinks, many authorities, impressed by studies that suggest the benefits of sports drinks in terms of performance and recovery, now recommend these drinks for shorter workouts as well. Remember, you can make your own rehydration drink by mixing one part fruit juice with one part water.

In addition to water and carbohydrates, you have to replace the electrolytes lost in sweat. A pound of sweat contains approximately 500 mg of sodium and 100 mg of potassium, and large fluid losses can be accompanied by substantial electrolyte losses. Sodium and potassium enhance fluid and glucose uptake, so you also need to replenish them during and after exercise.

Luckily, these electrolytes are readily found in food sources. Most sports drinks and foods contain adequate amounts of sodium and potassium to meet your needs.

Finally, although moderate use of alcohol the day before a competitive event doesn't appear to influence physical performance, several recent studies have shown that excessive drinking the evening prior to a competition may "elicit deleterious effects on performance the following morning." In other words, competing with a hangover isn't a good idea.

9

SUPPLEMENTATION IS NOT A SPORT

Vitamins and minerals are called micronutrients because we need very small amounts of them. Although they provide no direct source of energy, they insure effective metabolism, growth, and repair. As such, they are essential for life.

Vitamins are divided into two groups: those that are fat soluble (vitamins A, D, E, and K) and those that are water soluble (vitamin C and the B vitamins). Fat-soluble vitamins dissolve into the fat cells, where they can be stored. Because they can be stored, they may accumulate to toxic levels if taken in excess. Water-soluble vitamins, on the other hand, are rarely toxic, because the body can flush the excess amount out in the urine.

Minerals are also divided into two groups: the major minerals and the trace minerals, based on the quantity in which they are found in the body. As with fat-soluble vitamins, excessive amounts of minerals can be toxic and result in illness.

Because both deficient and excessive intakes of vitamins and minerals pose problems, it is important that you keep your intake within a safe range. That range is outlined by the Recommended Dietary Allowance (RDA) established by the Food and Nutrition Board of the National Academy of Sciences. The RDAs are the levels of essential nutrients currently thought to be adequate to meet the basic nutritional requirements of healthy individuals.

Micronutrient intakes of less than 70 percent of the RDA are considered deficient. Excessive intakes are generally defined as ten times the RDA, but in some instances can be less. For vitamin A, toxic symptoms occur at levels as low as five times the RDA; for vitamin D, at only twice the RDA. In excess, vitamins can begin acting more like drugs than nutrients.

Because the RDAs are broken down into 17 categories, there is no room to publish each category on a food label. For that reason, food and supplement labels list the micronutrients they contain as the percentage of the daily value (%DV), rather than as a percent of the RDA the nutrient contains. The %DV represents the highest value recommended for the nutrient. The recommendation for an adult male, for example, is 10 milligrams (mg) of iron each day. The recommendation for a premenopausal woman is 15 mg. No one else has as high a recommendation for iron. Therefore, the %DV is set for the woman, rather than the adult male.

The Confusion Surrounding the RDA

The RDAs are relied upon by food manufacturers and the general public as if they are fixed values, but in reality the RDAs are recommendations, rather than requirements for a specific individual. It is worth noting that the %DV is based on the highest level of RDAs for any particular group of healthy but sedentary adults. Children and infants are not even factored into the %DV. An individual's health status, activity levels, and an individual's genetics and history will also influence how much of any micronutrient a particular individual needs. And there is limited research to date on athletic populations, who conceivably may have different requirements than the general population.

Recent studies, for example, suggest that amounts of certain vitamins, minerals, and other nutrients above the RDAs may be necessary for optimal health or even normal functioning, especially if the individual is under stress or maintaining high levels of performance for prolonged periods of time. Vitamins C, E, and beta-carotene have been extensively studied at levels much higher than the RDA. Supplementation in megadose quantities of ten times the RDA, especially in combination, has been found to have potent antioxidant properties.

This is beneficial because antioxidants minimize the damage to cell membranes and other cellular components by free radicals, which are compounds thought to be involved in aging and the development of heart disease and cancer, the two leading causes of death in the United States. Of more immediate interest to the athlete, these antioxidants speed the repair process and minimize the muscle damage caused by exercise and environmental stressors such as smog and other pollutants.

Too Much Is Still Too Much

Even so, although most research points to little, if any, adverse effects of elevated antioxidant intake, many other micronutrients cannot make this claim. Any excessive amount of vitamin A may result in weakness, headache, nausea, joint pain, liver damage, and deformities to a developing fetus. Five times the RDA of vitamin D may lead to vomiting, diarrhea, loss of muscle tone, and soft tissue damage. Twice the RDA of niacin and vitamin B6 have been shown to, among other things, decrease athletic performance.

Several minerals have also demonstrated toxicity symptoms when taken in megadose quantities. Despite the common perception that we do not get enough iron in our diet, iron in higher amounts than the RDA can cause cirrhosis of the liver, an increased risk of colon cancer, elevated cholesterol levels, and an increased risk of heart disease. In excessive amounts, it can be fatal to young children. Therefore, only premenopausal women should consider an iron supplement during menses and should only do so with a doctor's recommendation. Because of this information, many supplement manufacturers have removed iron from products geared toward males and postmenopausal females. But many have not.

Other minerals that are toxic in excess include zinc, chromium, and selenium. Intakes of zinc at approximately six times the RDA may increase the risk of heart disease by elevating LDL cholesterol and decreasing HDL cholesterol levels. Although zinc lozenges have been shown to reduce the duration and severity of symptoms associated with the common cold, excessive amounts, particularly when taken orally in tablet form, actually decrease immune function. Although the National Research Council indicates that dietary chromium does not appear to be toxic, supplementation has been shown to cause chromosomal damage in laboratory animals, as well as behavior disorders in humans. Amounts greater than ten times the RDA of selenium, which is often regarded as an anticancer supplement, have been known to cause nausea, vomiting, abdominal pain, hair loss, and fatigue.

Getting What You Paid For

Overconsumption can not only be toxic, but can affect bioavailability, which is the term used to describe the degree to which the amount of an ingested nutrient is absorbed and available to the body. The bioavailability of many micronutrients (minerals in particular) varies based upon what nutrients are present in the digestive tract at the same time. Because an excess of one nutrient can dramatically affect the absorption of other nutrients, most nutritionists caution against randomly taking individual supplements unless warranted by a specific medical condition and under the guidance of a qualified health professional.

I agree with those nutritionists, particularly when we're speaking about the athletes I work with. They not only have a high caloric intake, but eat many foods that are fortified with many vitamins and minerals. Most energy bars and drinks, as well as many cereals, have these recommended micronutrients added at levels that are close to the RDA. Often an athlete will eat several servings during training alone. When it comes to cereal, some will eat the whole box as a normal serving size, rather than the recommended half-cup that typically contains 25 to 100 percent of the daily value for many of the key vitamins and minerals. For that reason, there's no reason to spend money and risk toxic side effects on unnecessary and potentially detrimental supplements.

Scientists have recently begun to investigate another category of nutrients called phytonutrients. There are literally thousands of these herbs, food enzymes, flavanoids, and other plant-derived compounds found in fruits, vegetables, and other plants that are essential for optimal health and that are useful in the treatment of a variety of diseases.

Although many of the plants that contain them have been used medicinally for thousands of years, particularly in Eastern medicine, many of these compounds have not been isolated. Some that have include isoflavones found in soy products, isothiocyanates and allyl sulfides in vegetables, and ferulic acid, caffeic acid, and limonene in fruits. Because hundreds of known, and as of yet unknown, chemicals are present in the fruits and vegetables we eat, it is much wiser to rely on foods as a source of a balanced supply of micronutrients than on a pill or tablet containing only one, or a few, of these nutrients.

Bioavailability is an issue with whole foods, as well as with supplements. The amount of a nutrient that is listed on a label or food chart may not be the actual amount you are getting. Vitamin losses occur during food processing, food storage, and preparation. Once a fruit or vegetable has been picked, the vitamin content immediately begins to diminish. Canning or other processing destroys even more of the nutrients. Improper shipping and storage that results in exposure of the food to heat, air, or light further reduces the quantity of vitamins in the food. Finally, prolonged cooking, excessive heat, and exposure to hot water lead to significant vitamin losses.

To make sure you are getting the most nutrients possible, it is always best to rely on local produce. Reduce your intake of processed foods, which inevitably destroy some of the nutrients, and eat fruits and vegetables in as raw or uncooked a state as possible.

If You Still Want To

After all is said and done, most athletes are still going to be willing guinea pigs for the latest supplement craze. This is because sports nutrition is not an academic subject to them, but is their lifeblood. Because they are so performance oriented, they are notoriously gullible in regard to fad products and anecdotal claims that promise to be the new magic bullet. That naivete makes athletes a marketing department's dream, and helps explain the steady stream of new "essential" supplements, and expensive performance-enhancement products that cram the pages of the fitness magazines and the shelves of the health-food stores.

As the information in this chapter shows, there is very little reason for healthy athletes who are not on calorically restricted diets to take anything more than a daily multi-vitamin and mineral supplement for insurance. Even so, many athletes still insist on supplementation. To determine if a product is worthwhile, remind yourself that many supplement manufacturers are in the business of making money rather than promoting health or increasing performance. Then take it upon yourself to research all the product's claims. You owe it to yourself to be as informed as possible.

To make sure that the product is safe and effective, find out whether controlled scientific studies have been performed on the product and whether these studies have produced enough credible scientific knowledge to suggest a benefit.

The evidence has to support safety *and* effectiveness—one is not good enough to warrant your taking the supplement. Certain micronutrients have been shown to be effective, but may have questionable long-term or even short-term side effects. Others may be safe, but have no effect on performance.

A lot of people, for example, are singing the praises of a nutrient called inosine. Despite a well-financed marketing campaign claiming that it is an ergogenic (performance-boosting) aid, several scientific studies have shown it to be detrimental to performance. Because it has not been shown to be effective, I certainly would not recommend it to my clients or take it myself.

Boron is another nutrient that is being oversold. It is an important trace mineral involved in bone metabolism and development. There is evidence that some women could benefit from taking it, particularly after menopause, but it is also being marketed as a natural testosterone booster. The research the manufacturers quote, however, studied the effects of nutrition on the bone development of postmenopausal women. There was no reference in the study to males, and no demonstrated increase over normal testosterone levels. Subsequent studies have also shown that there was no improvement in performance either. Since there is no evidence to support the marketing claims that persist to this day, there is no reason for men—or most women— to add a boron supplement to their diets.

As these examples prove, even if it takes some effort, you should read the studies that are being quoted. You can ask the manufacturer for copies of the scientific studies they based their claims on. If you don't have access to a research library, the Internet is an excellent source of information. Frequently, however, the information is unregulated and inaccurate. For safety's sake, rely on websites in the Resources section of this book, (page 263) or on websites that reference peer-reviewed research journals such as those listed in the resource list. These websites are among the most authoritative available. Others may seem objective, but may be funded by pharmaceutical companies or by other companies with ulterior motives.

Once you've decided to purchase a micronutrient supplement, whether in isolated form or in combination with other micronutrients, you can reduce your expense and increase the quality of your purchase by following a few simple tips:

First, to ensure freshness, only buy supplements that have an expiration date on them, and make sure you will be finished with the bottle several months before the expiration date.

Second, with the exception of natural vitamin E (d-alpha tocopherol, as opposed to the synthetic form dl-alpha tocopherol), do not worry about whether or not a product is natural. There is no difference between a natural and synthetic supplement other than cost.

Third, the difference in bioavailability between chelated minerals and nonchelated minerals is only 5 to 10 percent. That may only justify their expensive price tag if cost is not an issue to you.

Fourth, find out if each ingredient in the product meets or exceeds the United States Pharmacopia (USP) standards for purity. If the product does, it will have the letters *USP* on the label. This rating guarantees that the products meet the voluntary standard set for activity, quality, and the ability to dissolve as verified by an official testing bureau.

Top Hits

Although the list of substances used by athletes is continually expanding, some of the more commonly used nutritional supplements by athletes today include amino-acid supplements, antioxidants, bee pollen, boron, carbohydrate supplements, carnitine, chromium, coenzyme Q10, creatine, gamma-oryzanol, ginseng, glycerol, beta-hydroxy-beta-methylbutyrate (HMB), inosine, lecithin, medium-chain triglycerides, multivitamin-mineral supplements, pyruvate, vanadium, yohimbine, numerous vitamins and minerals and others. These nutritional supplements are legal for use by the International Olympic Committee (IOC) and other sports governing agencies and are readily available at the health-food store. Because they are so popular, it is worth looking at each individually.

Amino-acid supplements, individually or in combination, along with other protein supplements, are taken in the hopes of boosting blood levels of amino acids, and the anabolic hormones testosterone, growth hormone, or insulinlike growth factor I (IGF-I) to enhance endurance, reduce fatigue, aid recovery, improve strength, and increase muscle mass while decreasing body fat.

Taken individually, particularly in excess, amino acid supplements can be toxic and create imbalances of other amino acids in the body. For these reasons the FDA, in 1974, removed amino acids from its list of substances that are generally recognized as safe. The FDA-assigned panel of experts particularly warned against amino acid use in populations at high risk of suffering health problems as a result of ingesting amino-acid supplements. Those at risk include children and teenagers, pregnant and breast feeding women, pre-menopausal women, elderly and others with particular medical conditions.

To date, few scientific studies support the use of particular amino-acid supplements for performance enhancement or body-composition changes. Ingesting a diet of foods supplying adequate amounts of protein will meet all of your individual amino-acid requirements at a fraction of the cost of supplements and with no added health risks.

The branched-chain amino acids (BCAA), leucine, isoleucine, and valine, are essential nutrients that can easily be obtained in recommended levels by eating a typical diet including protein rich foods. Although they are present in large amounts in skeletal muscle, making up over 30 percent of all muscle protein, and are the main amino acids used by muscles for fuel, the amounts used are negligible compared to glucose and fatty acids. The only improvements in performance with amino-acid supplements are in endurance events where athletes will be competing for longer than three hours.

Protein supplements are taken by athletes to boost their overall protein intake. They do this in the mistaken belief of its stimulating muscle growth. While appropriate levels of protein are required for muscle growth, it is training that stimulates growth and repair. Any excess protein above your requirement is broken down and used for energy, stored as body fat, and the excess nitrogen is excreted by the kidney, putting an extra burden on the body and robbing the bones of precious calcium. While protein powders may be a convenient method of getting one's protein requirements, they are an expensive means. As long as you are taking in adequate calories it is unlikely a protein or complete amino-acid supplement is necessary to meet your protein needs.

Antioxidant supplements include the most common individual nutrients, vitamins C, E and beta-carotene (a precursor for vitamin A), selenium, and CoQ10, either taken individually or in combination. Numerous other antioxidants exist in foods, particularly fruits and vegetables, as well as being produced in the body. While studies have not found antioxidants to enhance performance, their main role may be involved in limiting some of the damage caused by exercise.

Antioxidant supplements may help bolster the body's natural defense mechanisms to oxidative stress. Exercise, particularly exhaustive and/or eccentric exercise, induces free radical formation and increases the level of oxidative stress. Free radicals damage cell membranes, membrane proteins and lipids, induce muscle soreness, and damage and limit recuperation. Although exercise increases the level of free radicals in the body, exercise also increases the levels of the body's own natural antioxidants, including superoxide dismutase, glutathione peroxidase, and catalase. Selenium, zinc, copper, and other trace minerals may exert their antioxidant affects through their incorporation into glutathione peroxidase and other enzymes, which protect cell membranes against free radical damage. Studies have shown that the amount of oxidative damage caused to DNA as a result of exhaustive exercise is significantly less in trained compared to untrained subjects.

Free radicals are highly toxic compounds generated naturally as a result of cellular metabolism as well as caused by numerous environmental agents such as cigarette smoke, smog, and ozone. They damage cell lipids and other compounds by oxidizing and modifying their structure. This oxidation process is believed to play a role in cell aging, heart disease, cancer, and other chronic, degenerative diseases. While the body produces natural antioxidants, there is much debate as to whether adequate amounts are produced or derived through dietary sources to meet the daily needs.

Although deficiencies in these antioxidants are uncommon, studies done on animals made deficient in one or more of these compounds have found decreases in performance. Animal studies on vitamin E–deficient animals have found greater amounts of oxidative damage on their cell membranes and earlier exhaustion times during exercise when compared to animals taking in normal levels of vitamin E. Vitamin E supplements resulted in reduced oxidative damage to muscle fibers and heart tissue caused by exercise.

Human studies on individual supplements and mixtures have found promising results. Three weeks of 200-mg vitamin E supplementation resulted in a reduction in postexercise markers of oxidative stress. A study performed using an antioxidant mixture of beta-carotene, vitamin C, and vitamin E found significantly lower levels of lipid peroxidation (representing oxidative damage) at rest and following exercise than in subjects not receiving supplementation.

While antioxidant supplementation may be warranted for athletes in amounts slightly higher than the RDA, it is important to remember that numerous other beneficial compounds are present in the foods we eat. These include the phytonutrients found in fruits and vegetables such as isoflavones in soy products, isothiocyanates found in broccoli, brussels sprouts, and cauliflower, allyl sulfides found in onions, garlic, and chives, and ferulic acid, caffeic acid, and limonene found in fruits. All of these phytonutrients help supply additional antioxidant compounds and have been shown to be beneficial in reducing cell damage and disease risk. Taking high levels (10 to 15 times the RDA) of individual antioxidants, such as vitamin C, may actually stimulate free radical damage. It has been long known that vitamin C can exert a pro-oxidant effect by stimulating free radical damage when it is placed in a test tube with iron or some other metals.

Bee pollen is collected from flowering plants and represents a mixture of vitamins, minerals, and amino acids. Each manufacturer's supplement varies from the source of plant used for production. While no specific nutrient within bee pollen has been shown to enhance performance, many athletes use it in the belief that the combination of "natural" ingredients will benefit their strength, endurance, and recovery.

Of all the studies performed using bee pollens from various sources, none have shown any benefits to muscular strength or endurance, cardiovascular endurance, or recovery. In addition, no mood enhancing or delay in fatigue has been found using bee pollen. A major concern with its use is the possibility of an allergic reaction, sometimes even life-threatening. Several case studies have reported serious adverse side effects from ingestion of bee pollen including headaches, nausea, diarrhea, and gastrointestinal distress along with anaphylaxis.

Boron is a nonessential trace mineral that is found in fruits, vegetables, and nuts. No RDA has been established for boron, which appears to play a role in normal bone development and mineralization. Boron deprivation is highly unlikely with a normal diet. Commercially available tablets are targeted to strength athletes as a means to increase muscle mass, decrease body fat, and to naturally raise testosterone levels.

Early research on postmenopausal women, who had been placed on a boron-deficient diet, showed enhanced calcium and magnesium metabolism, more favorable conditions for bone mineralization, and increased testosterone levels following reintroduction of boron into their diet. Based on more current research, several studies have shown that boron supplementation does not increase blood testosterone levels, muscle mass, strength, or fat loss in women or men who eat a typical diet, nor in body builders undergoing intense training. Based on the boron supplementation research, while safe at intakes of less than 10 milligrams per day, boron is not effective at raising natural testosterone levels, increasing muscle mass, or reducing body fat levels.

Carbohydrate supplements either in drink or solid form are a convenient way to provide essential nutrients during and after competition. In liquid form they not only provide essential nutrients for energy production but also help maintain blood volume and performance. Taken in solid form they are usually combined with other nutrients and supplements. While carbohydrates are one of the few nutrients that have conclusively been shown to be essential to performance and recovery, it is possible to obtain adequate amounts from dietary sources without the need for supplementation. With the exception of ultra-endurance athletes requiring highly concentrated forms of nutrients, all other athletes can obtain adequate amounts from foods and drinks taken during and after exercise without the need for supplementation. One particular consideration with carbohydrate supplementation is the gastrointestinal sensitivity to fructose and glucose polymers used in many sports supplements. While they are beneficial in terms of performance, many people can only tolerate limited amounts before experiencing diarrhea or other discomfort. Testing any supplement during training will help to avoid potential deleterious effects during competition.

Carnitine is a water-soluble, vitaminlike compound that facilitates the transport of long-chain fatty acids into the mitochondria. Carnitine plays other metabolic roles as well, which have been theorized to be performance enhancing. Although carnitine is an extremely important catalyst for metabolic reactions in muscle, it is not an essential dietary nutrient because it is formed from other nutrients in the liver from several amino acids. Carnitine is also found in substantial amounts in foods of animal origin, but is much lower in plant-based foods. Vegetarians tend to have lower levels of carnitine and may benefit from supplementation. Carnitine exists in two forms, D- and L-carnitine, and only the L-form can be utilized by the body. It is recommended to avoid D-carnitine, which may interfere with normal L-carnitine function.

Research results have been contradictory in terms of carnitine's effects on performance. Most studies have found no significant benefit from supplementation in terms of fuel utilization, lactic acid accumulation, acid-base balance, maximal aerobic capacity, anaerobic exercise capacity, recovery or performance in endurance activities. While L-carnitine supplementation has been shown to increase blood levels after a period of two weeks, little change is seen in muscle levels, where 95 percent of the bodies stores are found. Several studies have shown benefits in terms of reduced muscle damage and postexercise muscle soreness as well as improved exercise capacity in patients with serious diseases. Studies on carnitine supplementation for fat and weight loss have also been inconclusive. From the available research, it appears that while carnitine appears to be safe at levels up to six grams a day, its use is only recommended for vegetarians who may have low levels of carnitine.

Chromium is an essential mineral found naturally in foods, particularly whole grains, molasses, mushrooms, and asparagus. While no RDA for chromium exists, the Estimated Safe and Adequate Daily Dietary Intake (ESADDI) is 50 to 200 micrograms. Chromium is poorly absorbed in the intestinal tract, with less than 1 percent being absorbed with intakes within the ESADDI range. However, long-term intakes above the ESADDI level are not recommended because animal studies have shown chromosomal damage with long-term use and possible carcinogenic effects. Behavioral disorders have also been linked to excessive chromium levels because picolinate, a common component in chromium supplements, may adversely affect neurotransmitter functions in the brain. Another drawback of chromium supplementation is that excessive dietary intake inhibits zinc and iron absorption as well as decreasing blood iron stores. Several forms of chromium are available, including chromium picolinate, chromium polynicotinate, chromium chloride, and chromium-enriched yeast. Each are touted by their respective companies as being the most effective, but no evidence exists that there is any difference between the various forms.

Chromium's main function is as an essential component of the glucose-tolerance factor, which enhances insulin sensitivity. Therefore, chromium enhances the activity of insulin in transporting glucose out of the blood. Claims regarding increased lean muscle mass, decreased body fat stores, or increases in muscle strength are not confirmed by several scientific studies. Studies ranging from 6 to 14 weeks have shown no changes in body composition, fat loss, weight loss, muscle strength, aerobic endurance, or performance in both athletic and sedentary subjects. In fact, in one study on obese women, women who consumed 400 micrograms of chromium picolinate for nine weeks, actually gained a significant amount of weight rather than losing weight. From all of the above data and potential adverse side effects, the use of chromium for body composition or performance benefits seems questionable.

Coenzyme Q10 (ubiquinone) is a lipid-soluble compound that plays an integral role in metabolism as a component of mitochondrial metabolic pathways. It is found in highest concentrations in heart muscle and organ tissues. Coenzyme Q10 also functions as an antioxidant. Studies performed on diseased cardiac patients have found improved heart function, maximal aerobic capacity, and exercise performance when using coenzyme Q10 supplements.

While studies on heart patients appear promising, none of the well-controlled scientific studies using coenzyme Q10 supplements with healthy subjects have shown any performance benefits. Although numerous studies have reported increased blood levels of coenzyme Q10 following supplementation no improvements in maximal aerobic capacity, oxygen uptake, substrate utilization or performance were found. In fact, just the opposite has been noted in several studies. Increased levels of lipid peroxidation (or cell damage) were found in one study for the group taking coenzyme Q10 supplements, and in another the supplemented group had higher levels of markers for muscle damage. In another study, looking at coenzyme Q10's effects on performance, times for a simulated time trial race were significantly slower for the supplemented group compared to the placebo group. Many of these results may be due to the fact that when coenzyme Q10 is taken orally, it auto-oxidizes and actually produces free radicals and damages cells' mitochondria, thereby limiting cells' oxidative energy producing capabilities.

Creatine is a nitrogen containing organic compound that the body produces in limited amounts and is found almost exclusively in muscle. Because we only produce limited amounts, approximately one gram per day, optimal levels come from a diet containing animal protein sources because creatine is not found in plant foods. Commercially available powders are targeted to strength athletes as a means to increase muscle mass, increase muscle power, enhance anaerobic recovery, and decrease body fat. Adequate creatine is essential for maintaining normal levels of intramuscular creatine phosphate (CP). Creatine phosphate is an immediate energy source within the muscle used to resupply ATP stores and sustain a high energy output for explosive sports demanding power and speed such as short-distance running, football, volleyball, or those involving sprinting, jumping, lifting, and hitting.

Numerous studies have shown that oral creatine supplementation in amounts of 20 to 30 grams per day for five to seven days significantly raises intramuscular creatine and CP levels at rest and during recovery from exercise. Taking carbohydrates concurrently, at a level of 90 grams/five grams of creatine, will significantly enhance creatine storage. Elevated creatine levels are maintained for prolonged periods with a maintenance doses of two to three grams per day.

Creatine is one of the few supplements studied that has conclusively shown benefits on short-term power performance, increases in muscle mass, and increased muscle power during repetitive bouts of weight lifting. The increase in body weight seen with creatine use makes it detrimental for most endurance athletes, where an increase in body mass would increase energy requirements and reduce aerobic capacity. Creatine is not a significant energy source for long-term aerobic exercise.

Although creatine supplementation has been shown to be safe in both short-term and long-term studies, anecdotal reports indicate that increased muscle cramping may result in some individuals using creatine. Increasing fluid intake is generally recommended to combat any potential deleterious effects.

Gamma-oryzanol is a two-part molecule, a plant sterol (fat) combined with ferulic acid, which is extracted from rice bran oil. Many anabolic claims are made about plant sterols, although it appears that the active portion of gamma-oryzanol is found in the ferulic acid. One problem with gamma-oryzanol is its low bioavailability. Less than 10 percent of sterol is absorbed in the digestive tract, with much of it being degraded. When given in a liquid form this number goes up to 40 to 60 percent. Taking more of the product does not appear to raise the amount absorbed. Research into its performance enhancing actions is limited, however, it has been found to have a variety of physiological effects, one of which is a lowering of blood cholesterol levels.

Some of the performance claims surrounding gamma-oryzanol include increasing natural testosterone levels, stimulating the release of growth hormone, and as a result of these two effects, increasing muscle mass, decreasing body fat levels, and improving muscle strength and endurance.

To date, only one well controlled scientific study has looked into the efficacy of gamma-oryzanol for athletes. Following nine weeks of weight training there were no differences in body mass, body fat, muscular strength, or muscle power as measured by vertical jump tests in athletes taking gamma-oryzanol or a placebo. Both groups improved to the same degree, showing that gamma-oryzanol has no additional effect and that a properly designed training program will improve these parameters.

While gamma-oryzanol appears to be safe in low dosages and may have beneficial health effects, taking the supplement for performance enhancement does not seem warranted.

Ginseng is a plant whose extract has been promoted as an energy booster. Ginseng extracts contain the physiologically active chemical ginsenosides. The extract varies depending on the part of the plant used, the plant species, and the place of origin. Unfortunately, commercial products vary considerably in concentrations of the active compounds. In fact, in a recent survey by an independent laboratory, over 10 percent of the products contained no detectable levels of ginsenosides. Ginseng supplements have been studied to determine their effects on performance, particularly in regard to increased energy production from all three energy systems.

While several studies have shown ginseng to be beneficial for diabetic subjects in terms of blood-glucose regulation, no benefits have been found for healthy, athletic individuals. In several recent studies no performance enhancement was seen in oxygen uptake, lactic acid accumulation, heart rate, or ventilatory responses, running or cycling performance, nor mood or perceived exertion comparing ginseng groups to placebo. One additional concern for athletes involved in events where drug testing takes place is that several commercially available ginseng products also contain the banned substance ephedrine.

Glycerol is one of the by-products of triglyceride (fat) breakdown. Since glycerol can be converted into glucose in the liver, it is hypothesized to be an effective fuel source during exercise. Glycerol feeding during exercise, however, has not been shown to prevent either hypoglycemia (low blood glucose) or muscle glycogen depletion and therefore has no effect on muscle fuel metabolism.

A secondary effect of glycerol is in promoting fluid and water retention. Glycerol may therefore be used to increase body water stores, including blood volume, prior to exercise. This may prove valuable for improving cardiovascular function and body temperature regulation, particularly when competing in hot environments.

The hyperhydration effect of glycerol reduces the overall heat stress of exercise. Studies have shown that glycerol supplementation prior to exercise increases sweat rate, leads to a lower exercise heart rate and body temperature, as well as an enhancement in endurance performance. By reducing heat stress glycerol provides a measure of safety when competing in a hot, humid environment.

The typical preexercise recommendation is to ingest one gram of glycerol per kilogram of body weight along with one to two liters of water consumed one to three hours prior to competition. The effects last for up to six hours. No benefit is seen when consumed during exercise or when small quantities of water are consumed. Glycerol does come with potential side effects including nausea, dizziness, bloating, light-headedness, weight gain and headaches.

HMB (beta-hydroxy-beta-methylbutyrate) is a by-product of leucine metabolism in the body. Leucine is an amino acid normally obtained in any diet and is the normal source of HMB production in the body. HMB is found in varying quantities in dietary sources. Some rich sources include catfish and grapefruit. HMB has been proposed as increasing muscle mass, decreasing body fat, and limiting muscle breakdown during intense training.

Several short-term studies have found increases in lean body mass and muscle strength along with reduced body fat levels and markers of muscle damage. Among the most promising of the results were those showing reduced levels (20 to 60 percent lower than control) of indicators of muscle breakdown (proteolysis). These results found HMB to prevent or slow muscle damage and limit muscle breakdown resulting from intense resistance weight lifting. Such changes would allow for higher intensities of training and more rapid muscle repair.

Because all of the human studies on HMB thus far have been performed by one laboratory, the one that developed HMB, further research is needed to confirm these results. Long-term studies must be performed that look at the safety of chronic HMB ingestion.

No reports of side effects from intakes up to 4 grams per day for several weeks have been observed. The safety with long-term use in presently not known, although in animal studies no adverse side effects have been noted. If selecting a product for use, keep in mind that HMB is a patented product by Metabolic Technologies, Inc. (MTI). Although several HMB products exist on the market, only those products listing the patent number contain actual HMB.

Inosine is a nucleic acid derivative, unlike the advertised claims of it being an amino acid. The body produces adequate amounts of this nonessential nutrient from amino acids and glucose, although it can be found in foods such as brewer's yeast and organ meats. In the body, inosine helps to form adenosine, one of the structural components of ATP, the body's energy currency. Inosine supplementation is therefore proposed to enhance ATP production and levels. Other claims include inosine's ability to improve oxygen delivery to working muscles, improve endurance capacity, reduce lactic acid buildup, and enhance both anaerobic and aerobic exercise performance.

Unfortunately, this is not the case. Several studies have shown inosine supplementation to have no effect on any of the above parameters. In fact, two studies found inosine supplementation to significantly impair and reduce performance in both cyclists and runners when compared to placebo groups. Current scientific research does not support the use of inosine as an ergogenic aid.

Lecithin is the most common phospholipid in foods. It is found in significant amounts in wheat germ, soybeans, spinach, and cauliflower, along with higher fat foods such as nuts, organ meats, and egg yolks. Lecithin's primary function in the body is in fatty acid and cholesterol transport and utilization. It is also a component of many cells in the body. Lecithin is not an essential nutrient because the body can manufacture adequate amounts. One of the constituents of lecithin, choline, plays an important role as a component of acetylcholine, the neurotransmitter responsible for sending the signals from nerve cells of muscle cells initiating their contraction.

Lecithin has been marketed to increase both muscle power and endurance along with adding in body fat loss. Due to the presence of choline, lecithin has also been purported to reduce fatigue. All of the studies to date have failed to show any positive effects on performance, body composition, fatigue, or recovery. Because many high-carbohydrate, low-fat diets are limited in their amounts of choline or lecithin, some investigators have recommended supplementation for individuals with low dietary choline intakes.

Medium-chain triglycerides (MCTs) release saturated fatty acids with shorter chain lengths (6 to 12 carbons). Being water soluble enables them to be absorbed directly into the blood without being converted into chylomicrons. They are transported directly to the liver and other tissues, where they generally undergo oxidation for energy production rather than storage as body fat. Because of their use primarily for energy production and their rapid processing, MCTs have been theorized to enhance endurance performance by increasing the contribution of fat for energy production and sparing muscle glycogen. They have also been marketed as increasing fat metabolism, increasing energy levels, and promoting fat loss and weight loss. Consuming MCTs does not impair gastric emptying as do common dietary fats. Although the MCTs enter the bloodstream very rapidly and increase blood levels of ketones (an indicator of fat catabolism) no changes in the metabolic fuel mixture have been noted at rest or during exercise. Both fats and carbohydrates are used in the same relative amounts. In fact, during exercise, MCT catabolism has been shown to only contribute between 3 and 7 percent of the total exercise energy cost.

During performance, several studies have shown negative effects with MCTs alone compared to placebo or carbohydrate ingestion. A recent study with cyclists found similar results of MCT use. When used alone during a 40-km time trial, the group who replaced carbohydrates with MCTs had an impaired performance of 8 percent. This detriment was similar to that found in earlier studies. Combining MCTs with carbohydrates yielded a 2.5 percent improvement compared to the carbohydrate-only group. The results of this one study have not been duplicated and more research is needed before conclusive support of MCT use is recommended.

MCTs provide little benefit when consumed with carbohydrates and impair performance when used alone, they often result in gastrointestinal distress such as cramping and diarrhea, so the use of MCTs is questionable. The ability to tolerate their use during exercise surely must be tested prior to competition.

Multivitamin-mineral supplements are often taken at RDA levels or above, sometimes at megadose quantities (1,000 percent or higher of the RDA) in hopes of protecting athletes from deficiencies and to enhance performance. Most typical one-a-day type supplements contain 100 percent of the RDA for most vitamins and minerals. Initially these one-a-day supplements were produced as insurance for diets with inadequate intakes of certain nutrients. For this purpose these serve their role well.

Vitamins and minerals act as coenzymes and cofactors for many enzymes involved in the metabolic reactions of the body, but in and of themselves they do not give us energy. Numerous other functions exist that theoretically could enhance cellular function and therefore athletic performance. In fact, studies have shown that when actual deficiencies do exist, taking a particular nutrient in supplement form will improve function and performance. Most individuals, however, are not deficient in most micronutrients.

Several long-term studies, lasting up to eight months, have looked at the effects of multivitamin-mineral supplementation on athletic performance. With dosages ranging from 100 to 5,000 percent of the RDA, no improvements in strength, endurance, or performance were seen. Most authorities agree that there is no need for supplementation for athletes who consume a balanced diet in both calories and nutrients. Taking a low-dosage, one-a-day type supplement for protection will benefit those athletes whose diets are restrictive in nutrient balance or calories.

It is also important to remember that many of the sports supplements, meal replacements, energy bars, as well as cereals and other foods, eaten by athletes are commonly fortified and supply the athlete with significant amounts of most essential micronutrients.

Pyruvate and Dihydroxyacetone (DHA) are both three-carbon intermediaries of carbohydrate metabolism. They are used in conjunction with one another in supplements and in scientific studies. They are found in fruits and vegetables, particularly apples. They have both been found to augment muscle glycogen content, and therefore would theoretically enhance endurance performance. They are also marketed to enhance fat loss.

While few studies have been performed using pyruvate and dihydroxyacetone, the combination of these supplements has produced significant improvements in aerobic endurance and reductions in perceived exertion. The improvements in both upper and lower body endurance were as high as 20 percent. The amounts used in the study were 100 grams (a 1:3 ratio with 25 g pyruvate and 75 g DHA). Most manufacturers recommend daily dosages of from two to five grams taken throughout the day. This is dramatically less than that used in the research studies and while at levels that are affordable, are questionable in terms of results. Pyruvate supplementation has also been shown to increase pre-exercise muscle glycogen levels when combined with a diet adequate in carbohydrates. This effect would benefit high-intensity endurance exercise to a similar extent as glycogen loading or carbohydrate ingestion during exercise.

The use of pyruvate has been found to enhance weight loss and body fat loss when used by obese individuals on extremely energy (calorie) restrictive diets. A group of obese women in a metabolic hospital ward taking 36 grams of pyruvate (representing 13 percent of the calories ingested per day) along with a 1,000 calorie diet containing 68 percent carbohydrate, 22 percent protein and 10 percent fat, lost 37 percent more weight (13.0 lb vs 9.5 lb) and 50 percent more fat (8.8 lb vs 5.9 lb) after three weeks than a group taking a placebo. While the exact mechanism for the effects of pyruvate are unknown, more research in this area is certainly warranted. The adverse side effects of high dosages of these supplements—those levels used in these studies—include gastrointestinal distress and diarrhea. Long-term safety and use are also still unknown. For weight loss and long-term maintenance, following a balanced diet along with exercise and lifestyle modification is the preferential recommendation over short-term restrictive dieting with rapid weight loss and the use of supplementation.

Vanadium is a nonessential trace mineral found in shellfish, grains, and pepper. Vanadium supplements are available as vanadium salts, primarily vanadyl sulfate. Vanadium exhibits insulinlike properties by facilitating glucose transport and glucose utilization in skeletal muscle along with increased glycogen synthesis. Using animal studies extrapolated to humans, proponents of its use suggest vanadyl to have an anabolic effect on muscle by inhibiting protein breakdown during exercise.

Studies on performance have shown vanadyl sulfate to have no effects on body fat, lean body mass, or strength performance during weight lifting. In human studies with noninsulin-dependent diabetics, dosages of 100 milligrams per day for four weeks were given and found to improve glucose tolerance. The safe use of larger dosages or for longer periods of time is unknown. Typical dosages taken by athletes using supplements are in the range of 20 to 60 milligrams. Side effects include diarrhea and gastrointestinal distress. However, excess supplementation may cause liver and kidney damage. These side effects, along with the limited positive research on vanadium, question its use as a dietary supplement.

Yohimbine is derived from the bark of yohimbine trees. It has druglike actions as an antagonist to epinephrine (adrenalin) at the receptor level. The primary effect is to increase production of epinephrine and has been used in the treatment of male sexual dysfunctions. Claims for its use include increasing testosterone levels, decreasing body fat, and stimulating muscle growth.

While one study found an increase in fat levels in the blood following yohimbine ingestion, no studies have found yohimbine to increase testosterone levels, decrease body fat, or alter body composition. The studies using yohimbine have reported numerous side effects including acute elevations in blood pressure, gastrointestinal distress, headache, dizziness, and shakes.

Magic Bullet? Quality of Research

While only some of the many nutritional sports supplements have been covered here, numerous other supplements and pharmaceutical agents exist that may or may not positively affect performance. More research is needed to determine their efficacy and safety. Many ergogenic (performance enhancing) substances, including pharmaceuticals, are banned for use by the International Olympic Committee (IOC). These and others are beyond the scope and focus of this review.

Once again, I caution you to remember that first and foremost supplement companies are in business to make money. Also be wary of information promoted in magazines or the Internet, because much of the information is misleading, overstated, or false. Beware the hype and check for scientific substantiation of the claims.

PART III

TRAINING SMART: THE ATHLETE'S HANDBOOK

BASIC TRAINING

The focus of *Fuel Up* is on sports nutrition, not on athletic training. However, just as many people think they are eating correctly yet are not, many people believe their workouts are more effective than they really are. While *Fuel Up* is not a book on training, it will help you understand the dynamics of exercise, particularly in relation to nutrition, so that your exercise becomes as efficient as your diet.

Many athletes and fitness enthusiasts alike overtrain or train improperly for their desired goals. Fitness encompasses many broad categories including cardiorespiratory fitness, muscular strength and endurance, flexibility, agility, and even body composition. This chapter will outline the basic principles of fitness. Chapters 11 and 12 will deal with more advanced goals and athletic performance.

Exercise Overload

Exercise is a stress that, when used properly, forces the body to adapt and become fitter. Like any stress, when done in excess it will cause the body and the mind to rebel. For that reason, the workouts in this chapter will be of a moderate intensity and duration. That will keep the goal of becoming fit realistic and will make sure that the workouts are not self-defeating.

Fuel Up adheres to the guidelines for exercise prescription established by the American College of Sports Medicine (ACSM), a prominent organization involved in scientific research and education in the areas of sports and exercise as they relate to health, fitness, performance, and disease prevention. These guidelines for cardiovascular and musculoskeletal fitness were established to develop levels of fitness for the general population based on the current scientific literature. While they won't develop blazing speed or maximal strength, they will provide the necessary stimulus for improvements in endurance, strength, and body composition.

Before we get into the specific guidelines, we need to reintroduce the concept of exercise overload. Exercise overload, which measures the amount of stress the exercise program is placing on the body, is composed of three variables: intensity (how hard you are working), duration (how long), and frequency (how many days per week). The following equation gives you an indication of your weekly training load:

Intensity (in calories/minute) × Duration (minutes/workout) × Frequency
(workouts/week) = Exercise Overload (calories/week).

Because fitness is an ongoing concern, these measurements should be taken weekly. When developing a workout program, concentrate on exercise overload as a whole, rather than on one particular variable or workout.

How Hard Are You Working?
Cardiovascular Conditioning

Of the three parameters, frequency and duration are fairly straightforward. Intensity, or the measure of how hard you are working, is less self-explanatory. The intensity of cardiovascular activities is based on your exercise heart rate. Monitoring your heart rate is one of the most accurate methods for calculating the intensity of your cardiovascular workout. Guidelines for exercise intensity are given as a percentage of your maximal heart rate (HRmax) (the target range being from [55–64 percent or 65–90 percent]). Other measures used to calculate exercise intensity are based on a percentage of heart rate reserve and maximal oxygen uptake (advanced techniques relevant to competitive athletes are covered in Chapter 20) or your rating of perceived exertion (RPE).

To calculate the intensity of your workout using maximal heart rate, first find out what your age-predicted HRmax is by subtracting your age from 220. Then, to determine how hard you should be working, multiply that number by 65 percent to obtain the lower level of your target heart rate zone (or, if you are unfit, 55–64 percent HRmax) and by 90 percent to obtain the upper limit of the training sensitive zone (high-intensity exercise). A 30-year-old, for example, would have a training intensity range for cardiovascular exercise from 124 to 171 beats per minute (220 − 30 years = 190 × .65 = 124 or 190 × .90 = 171). The table below lists age-appropriate exercise heart rate zones.

TARGET HEART RATE ZONE

AGE	LOWER LIMIT (65% HRmax)	UPPER LIMIT (90% HRmax)	Age-predicted HRmax
20	130	180	200
25	127	176	195
30	124	171	190
35	120	167	185
40	117	162	180
45	114	158	175
50	111	153	170
55	107	149	165
60	104	144	160
65	101	140	155
70	98	135	150
75	94	131	145
80	91	126	140
85	88	122	135
90	85	117	130

To monitor your exercise heart rate, you can either use a heart rate monitor or lightly place your middle and index finger on your radial pulse (located on the underside of the wrist). Don't bother taking your pulse during the warm-up, which is the first five to ten minutes of a workout, and during which you gradually reach your workout pace. Once you're warmed up, take your heart rate to see where you are relative to your target heart rate. Count each beat for 10 seconds, and multiply that number by 6. Then compare the number with your range of exercise intensity as indicated in the table above. Then take your pulse every 15 to 20 minutes during the workout or whenever you feel your intensity has dropped below or surpassed your target heart rate zone.

An easier way to gauge your effort is with your breath. If you can carry on a normal conversation with no difficulty at all, you are probably not working out hard enough. If you're gasping for breath, you're close to your max. If you can carry on a slightly labored conversation, you're probably within the lower reaches of your training heart rate.

Because it is simpler, most people use this method, if they use any method at all. It is not, however, as accurate as taking your pulse because you are not measuring how hard the body is working. To make the most of your workout, therefore, it is recommended that you take your pulse several times throughout your workout, especially if you are just beginning a fitness program.

Muscular Conditioning

The second component of fitness is muscular strength, which is developed with weight training or resistance exercise. These strength-conditioning guidelines concern themselves with muscular strength, weight management, and the ratio of lean body mass to body fat. While you burn significantly more calories during an aerobic workout than during a weight workout, the weight workout will have a greater overall effect on the calories you burn in a day. Because lean body mass is the primary contributor to your BMR (the number of calories you expend at rest) and weight workouts help to maintain or increase your lean body mass, they have a significant effect on your BMR because they not only burn calories during the weight workout, but also elevate your metabolism and the number of calories you burn the rest of the day and night.

You can see the difference body composition makes by comparing two 120-pound women. One has 10 percent body fat and the other 20 percent. The woman with 10 percent body fat has 108 pounds of lean muscle mass and 12 pounds of fat; the woman with 20 percent body fat has only 96 pounds of muscle and 24 pounds of fat.

One pound of lean muscle burns as much as ten times as many calories at rest a day as a pound of fat. Since one pound of muscle burns approximately 35 calories more than one pound of fat, the leaner woman can eat 420 more calories than the woman with the higher percentage of body fat can before gaining weight.

Strength Training Zone

Like endurance exercise, weight training also has an optimal training zone. Weight lifting intensity is measured by how much you lift and how many times you can do that lift. The number of times you perform a movement is called a repetition or rep. How much you lift per rep can be gauged by a term called your repetition maximum, or RM, and is based upon the maximal amount you can lift. Your 1RM is the maximal amount of weight you can lift with proper form. It corresponds to 100 percent of your capacity.

Science Matters

Studies have found a relationship to exist between %RM and number of reps an individual can perform. The relationship is as follows: 1RM = 100%RM, 3RM = 90%RM, 8RM = 80%RM, 12RM = 70%RM and 20RM = 60%RM. For example, if an individual can perform a 1RM on the barbell curl with 100 pounds, his 12 RM weight would be 70 pounds (or 70% of 100 lb). With a 70-pound barbell, the individual should be able to perform 12 repetitions with proper form.

The optimal range of repetitions for improvements in muscle strength, power, or size is from 60 percent to 100 percent of 1RM. This corresponds to a repetition range of 20 reps down to one. Training outside of this rep range will not be as effective at improving muscle function. In other words doing 12 repetitions with a very light weight is possible, but not effective unless that weight is the maximal amount you can handle for those twelve repetitions (i.e., a 12RM set).

The intensity guidelines for resistance training are based on the RM range. Because the procedure for determining RM is somewhat complicated, it is used primarily by competitive athletes. Most others use trial and error.

For general fitness one set of one exercise for each of the major muscle groups of the body is recommended. This set should conform to the eight-12RM range. Additional sets are utilized in advanced workouts geared to athletes. A resistance-training circuit usually takes between 20 and 30 minutes. You need two to three of these workouts, separated by at least 48 hours, per week. To reduce the risk of injury to the muscles, tendons, and joints, older or untrained individuals are encouraged to use lighter weights and higher repetitions.

The guidelines are the same whether you use free weights or

To Lose Weight, Stay Out of the Pool

Surprisingly, the one activity that most people trying to lose weight should avoid is swimming. In a landmark study performed at the University of Southern California, swimming was found to be unlike other forms of cardiovascular exercise because it doesn't result in significant loss of body fat or weight compared to land-based activities. We don't know exactly why that is, but it is suspected that higher levels of body fat are preferred for buoyancy and temperature regulation. Additional studies have shown that female swimmers have lower bone density than nonswimmers. For losing weight and maintaining or increasing bone density, then, weight-bearing activities appear to be more effective than swimming.

Swimming is, however, excellent for rehabilitation. If your physical condition limits you to swimming, by all means get in the pool. But if you are interested in losing weight or if you are worried about osteoporosis, it is imperative to incorporate some weight-bearing resistance training into your workout as well. As always, of course, be careful to work within your physical limitations.

machines. If you are not familiar with weight training, machines are easier to learn, don't require balance, and, at least in the beginning, are probably less intimidating than free weights. Free weights, on the other hand, mimic the movements of daily life and of sports, improve balance, and don't restrict you to a single plane of motion. You don't have to use one or the other; a combination of both allow for a variety of options.

Perhaps the best way to learn how to lift weights is by working with a qualified personal trainer. Be forewarned, however, that qualified trainers are not always easy to find. They should be certified by a reputable organization. The best of these are the ACSM, the

National Strength Conditioning Association (NSCA), and the American College of Exercise (ACE).

If you can't afford or can't find a trainer, start with basic exercises and simple movements. Your health club or gym probably has posters emphasizing proper form. Machines are required to have clear instructions for proper use on them, so read each set of instructions before you use them. Start with light weights that you can take through the entire range of motion.

If you are using free weights, also begin with weights that are light enough for you to handle comfortably. Think about how your joints move and let the movement with the weight recreate that pattern. If you are doing a bicep curl, for instance, drop your hands to your sides. You'll notice that your palm naturally turns into your thigh. Then, as you curl it up, it naturally rotates so that your palm faces your shoulder when your elbow is fully flexed. Adding a weight should not affect that range of motion or positioning. (This process does not work with barbells or other equipment because these alter the natural range of motion and the initial hand positions.)

Flexibility Conditioning: Flexibility and the Cooldown

Flexibility is defined as the range of motion possible around a joint or group of joints. Although flexibility is an integral component of fitness, many conditioning programs only pay lip service to it. This is unfortunate because improved flexibility and a broader range of motion can reduce the risk of injury, speed recovery, improve overall fitness, and enhance athletic performance. In its most recent guidelines on fitness and conditioning, the ACSM has included recommendations on flexibility training along with cardiovascular and musculoskeletal conditioning for developing overall health and fitness.

Improved flexibility can be achieved through three common stretching techniques: static stretches, dynamic stretches, and proprioceptive neuromuscular facilitation (PNF). Although each is effective, some carry a higher risk of injury than others.

While light stretching is often part of a warm-up, flexibility training is primarily performed during the final phase of the cooldown, when the muscles and connective tissue are adequately prepared for the stresses inherent in the stretches.

Static flexibility refers to joint mobility without regard to the speed of movement. True to their name, static stretches lengthen the muscle slowly and systematically by being held for at least 10 to, more effectively, 20 to 60 seconds. Because it produces the least amount of muscle tension, it is the technique best suited to the general public.

Dynamic flexibility involves increasing range of motion while the muscles and joints are actually moving. Athletes in sports or activities requiring rapid movement, such as gymnastics, football, tennis, golf, dancing, and the like, develop a certain amount of dynamic flexibility merely by participating in the activity. Because it has an inherent risk of injury, this method of flexibility training is only recommended for elite adult athletes working with a qualified coach or trainer. Most flexibility training regimens therefore concentrate on static stretching or controlled dynamic stretching such as yoga and tai chi, which enhances the range of motion, preferring to develop ballistic flexibility over time through participation in the actual activity.

Proprioceptive neuromuscular facilitation (PNF), which was originally developed for rehabilitative settings, incorporates a static stretch with an isometric contraction and relaxation (contract/relax). This is followed either by an additional static stretch or a second contraction. While there is conflicting data as to the effectiveness of PNF relative to static stretching, most experts believe the two are equally effective. Although PNF appears to be better at increasing the functional range of motion and flexibility where there are limitations (or areas of restricted movement), it is more difficult to learn and usually requires personalized instruction.

While stretching for as little as 10 seconds can improve flexibility, the most significant results can be achieved by holding the stretch for 20 to 60 seconds. If you don't have the time or patience to hold a stretch for a minute, try to hold each for 30 seconds. It is best to perform at least one stretch for each muscle, or muscle group, of the body even if your training does not involve all the muscle groups. Make sure to include a stretch for muscles on each limb, or side of the body as well. You can expect noticeable improvements in your flexibility in as little as three weeks by stretching two to three times a week.

Incorporating flexibility training into your routine does not require extensive equipment or a lot of space. You can do it on the floor in front of the television following your workout or while you are meditating and collecting your thoughts of the day. Because most of us tend to bypass flexibility training, you probably will have the most success in a stretching or a yoga class. Many people love yoga because it improves their flexibility without the monotony of basic repetitive stretches and because it has a soothing, supportive atmosphere.

Working Out As Meditation

Because many aerobic activities require relatively low skill and are repetitive in nature, they tend to be hypnotic, meditative right-brain activities that encourage creativity. Personally speaking, I derived inspiration for much of this book from my morning runs. Although I prefer to exercise in the morning as a way of getting started, other people may like to work out later in the day as a way to unwind. It doesn't matter when or how you exercise, as long as you lose yourself in movement. Once you do, you can achieve a spiritual balance that might otherwise be lacking in your life and simultaneously build daily activity into a previously inactive lifestyle. Because most people are sedentary, traditional meditative techniques, however spiritually beneficial, compound their lack of activity.

Most stretch and yoga classes are not intimidating, but like any type of group activity, make sure you attend the appropriate level class. Also, remember that the degree of flexibility around a joint or joints is limited by your anatomical structure, including your muscle mass and the connective tissue, your genetics, and your state of conditioning. Concentrate on improving your flexibility rather than on achieving some impossible ideal or competing with other people in the room.

The Basic Guidelines

Using the three parameters of exercise overload, the ACSM has developed the following basic guidelines for cardiovascular and muscular fitness:

OVERLOAD PARAMETER	CARDIOVASCULAR FITNESS GUIDELINES	MUSCULAR FITNESS GUIDELINES
EXERCISE FREQUENCY	3 to 5 days per week	2 to 3 days per week
EXERCISE DURATION	20 to 60 minutes	1 set of 8 to 10 exercises
EXERCISE INTENSITY	55/65%–90% of maximum heart rate (HRmax)	8 to 12RM if < 50 years 10 to 15RM if > 50 years

ACSM position stand. *Medicine and Science in Sports and Exercise* 30(6): 975–991, 1998.

Recently, the ACSM also incorporated guidelines for developing flexibility. These include performing stretching exercises for the major muscle groups of the body at least two to three times per week. Stretching can either be static or dynamic and can be performed in a group setting utilizing yoga or other forms of flexibility training.

How To Develop A Workout Program

The first step in planning an exercise program is realistically deciding how much time you can devote to exercise and how fit you are. To achieve cardiovascular fitness, you have to use aerobic activities that involve rhythmic movement and the major muscle groups of the body. Someone who can't handle a 20-minute workout can accumulate up to 60 minutes of 10-minute miniworkouts. For those who can, duration is dependent upon the intensity of the workout. The lower the intensity of the activity, the longer it needs to be performed.

Because fitness is a long-term proposition, it is best to begin with moderate intensity exercise of longer duration. Only when you begin training for athletic competition should you consider very high-intensity workouts. Several studies in the Department of Physiologic Science at the University of California at Los Angeles have shown that untrained individuals can get similar cardiovascular benefits from training below their target heart rate zone as they do from training at the high end of their zone—if the exercise overload, or the product of intensity times duration, remains the same. This means that those who cannot maintain the activity at intensities within their training sensitive zone throughout the workout will still benefit from it. Trained athletes, however, require higher intensity workouts to improve their fitness and performance.

Ideally, five to six workouts a week is most effective. This would include not only five to six 20 to 60 minute cardiovascular workouts, but also two to three weight training and flexibility workouts each week. If you can only spend three days a week working out, it is best to schedule at least three 60 to 90 minute cardiovascular workouts, at least one of which is followed by a strength training workout to satisfy your aerobic and caloric expenditure needs. Your flexibility training can be done during the cooldown.

If you're limited to 30 to 45 minutes before or after work or during lunch, plan on spending at least five days on aerobics. (Don't forget that you'll also have to add two to three half-hour weight resistance training workouts.)

To succeed over time, especially if you aren't used to exercise, you'll have the most success with an activity that you enjoy and that fits in the most with your lifestyle. If you don't know where to start, figure out what suits your personality and your needs. If you like camaraderie or are worried about your lack of discipline, begin with a group-oriented activity, such as an exercise class or hiking club. If you can afford it, hire a personal trainer. If you want more private time, gravitate toward solo sports such as running or cycling.

Do not cheat yourself by skipping your weight workouts, because they are your only real option in terms of building lean body mass in order to make your body's metabolism more efficient. Make sure to schedule two to three weight training workouts a week. These workouts can be done at the gym, using free weights and machines, or at your home, using home exercise equipment or containers such as milk cartons filled with sand. To reduce the risk of strain or injury, always use a weight you are comfortable with. It shouldn't be so light that you can lift it with no effort, or so heavy that is too painful to lift without control and proper form. Using higher repetitions and lighter weights is safer, particularly if you are just learning how to handle the weights.

Small Steps Win the Race

Regardless of how you choose to move, one benefit of regular exercise is that, as Julia Cameron writes in the book, *The Artist's Way*, "it teaches the sense of satisfaction over small tasks well done." Sometimes when you start working out, you feel overwhelmed and don't know how you'll get through it. Then, as you warm up and ease into the session, you relax with the process and feel a sense of confidence, knowing that you'll be able to complete it.

These concepts can be used on a larger scale. Starting a weight loss or exercise training program can be intimidating because making so many changes seems so insurmountable. But when you break the effort down into a series of small, predictable, and therefore manageable steps, you have a map and a structure that provide a sense of direction that guides you toward the larger goal.

Maintenance of Adaptation

Maintaining your fitness level during vacations or breaks from training during the off-season is always a concern. So is knowing what to do when you have reached a desired level of fitness or when you are overscheduled. Don't worry about losing that hard-earned conditioning. You can stay at your current level of fitness even though you don't have the same amount of time to devote to your workouts.

Scientific studies show that training intensity is more critical than duration and frequency, the other variables of exercise overload, in terms of maintaining fitness levels. Once you've attained a given fitness level, you can reduce exercise duration or frequency by up to two-thirds with no loss to conditioning for several months or longer. Of course, the other benefits of training, including emotional and weight control, may not be maintained or derived from these reduced volumes of training.

High-Intensity Training Adaptations

You cannot maintain high-intensity training consistently and not expect to have a setback. Just as it is important to give adequate recovery following a workout, it is also important to vary the intensity from workout to workout and from week to week. Periodization, or varying your workouts within a period of time, be it a week, month, or year, will allow you to continue to improve as well as peak for specific competitions. Cycle your training on a monthly basis so you alternate two or three weeks of relatively high-intensity periods of exercise with an easy week.

Home Exercise Equipment: Let the Buyer Beware

According to the National Sporting Goods Association, Americans spent three billion dollars on home fitness equipment in 1996. This is more than double the amount purchased just five years earlier. Now there's a huge market in used exercise equipment because people buy something that looks good in an ad but that they hate to use. Because so many of these machines end up as dust catchers or in garage sales, don't feel that you need the expensive toys for your resistance or, for that matter, your cardiovascular workouts.

Furthermore, many of the claims made for these machines are often misleading. There is no one machine that is best. Consider what you enjoy, what you find comfortable, what your goals are, what you can afford, and what kind of space you have. Then, before you buy the equipment, make sure you read the disclaimers and the fine print carefully.

Three words on those "miracle" abdominal machines that are advertised in magazines and on television: They don't work. Over the years my colleagues and I have tested dozens of the latest popularly advertised abdominal machines only to find that none were more effective than performing an abdominal crunch. And the beauty of an abdominal crunch is that it is free.

These guidelines are enough to keep you athletic throughout your life. They are not intense enough to provide optimal sports conditioning, but they do provide an adequate level of fitness so that you can smoothly move into more intense training if you want.

11

BOOT CAMP: TRAINING FOR STRENGTH AND APPEARANCE

Athletes lift weights to either improve their appearance or their performance, and they gear their training to develop muscle strength, size, and/or power. The distinctions are important because the goals are sports specific. Endurance athletes and those in weight-restricted sports such as boxing or wrestling and appearance-subjective sports such as gymnastics, figure skating, or diving want to improve their strength without adding muscle or additional weight to their bodies. Other athletes in sports such as bodybuilding want to increase the size of their muscles for appearance. And athletes who participate in racquet sports, golf, basketball, and other sports requiring explosive power want to improve their muscle power.

Reps and Sets

There are as many weight-lifting programs as there are trainers. One common flaw among most of these programs is the excessive nature of the workout. There is a tendency in weight rooms to push to the point of pain, but here, as in every other aspect of training, it is important not to overtrain. The rule is to elicit the appropriate stimulus for change, rather than an excessive amount that often leads to stagnation and frustration.

While the guidelines for minimal muscular fitness are one set per exercise and one exercise per body part, multiple sets and exercises yield greater results. Both anecdotal evidence and current research demonstrates that there is a significant increase in muscle strength when performing three sets per exercise compared to one or even two.

Would more than three sets of an exercise per body part be of benefit? For athletes seeking to improve their performance, the answer is yes. But while more sets are better, there is an upper limit. Multiple sets yield greater results, but the increased benefit from each additional set becomes smaller and smaller. This has much to do with the body's ability to handle the stress of the workout and its ability to recover. Because workouts with multiple sets take longer, time also becomes a consideration.

The guidelines for the total number of sets are from 8 to 12 sets for small muscle groups such as the biceps and deltoids, and 10 to 15 sets for large muscle groups, such as the quadriceps and the back. Warm-up sets will be performed for each exercise per body part, so the total number of RM sets will be less.

In terms of the number of repetitions for strength and power development, you need rep max sets in the range of 3–8 RM or at an intensity of 80–90 percent of your max. Athletes training for an increase in muscle size or endurance athletes who use weight training to improve performance require more repetitions, in the range of

12–20 rep max sets. This corresponds to an intensity level of approximately 60 to 70 percent of their max.

Recovery

The length of time you should rest between sets depends on what kind of training you are doing. An adequate rest period is generally anywhere from one to three minutes. The optimal rest period between rep max sets is three minutes, which allows for the muscle's energy sources to be replenished. Athletes interested in increasing their muscular endurance can gradually decrease the recovery time between rep max sets to one minute.

Frequency is another common concern. Training each muscle group twice per week is optimal. Athletes who lift weights four to six days per week must split up their muscle groups so that each muscle group is worked only twice per week. Only one of those workouts should be heavy; the other at a moderate level, without rep max sets, to allow for active recovery. Generally allow two to three days between workouts for the same muscle groups.

What You Get Is What You Want

Depending on your goals, you will want to train for strength, size, or power. Endurance athletes, anyone training for a toned appearance or base conditioning, and athletes like football players will all be interested primarily in strength because it will allow their muscles to generate more force. Bodybuilders, basketball centers, football linemen, some hockey players, shot putters and other field athletes are interested primarily in size. And sprinters, anyone involved in racquet sports, baseball players, golfers, gymnasts, divers, dancers, and anyone who needs rapid, explosive force are going to be interested primarily in power.

The type of adaptation required will determine how you train, including the type of muscle contraction and the speed at which it is performed. Athletes interested in size or power should begin a strength training program at least six to eight weeks prior to the sport-specific training. This develops an adequate musculoskeletal base of condition and reduces the risk of injury.

Muscle Contractions

When lifting a weight, there are two phases or types of muscle contraction. The first is a concentric contraction, in which the muscle shortens as the weight is being lifted. The other is an eccentric muscle contraction, in which the muscle lengthens as it develops force to resist either gravity or momentum. Whenever you lower a weight slower than gravity would move it, your muscles are performing an eccentric contraction.

Scientific studies have shown that muscles can generate 20 to 40 percent more force in the eccentric phase than in the concentric phase of contraction. This means that if you can lift 100 pounds for a 1RM biceps curl, you could lower 120 to 140 pounds during the eccentric phase of the movement. Because 120 pounds is greater than your concentric 1RM, you would need help getting the weight to the top position before you lowered it back down (a negative rep).

Because research has shown that these eccentric contractions are critical for developing muscle size, doing forced reps (for which you need assistance during the concentric phase of the final two or three reps of a set) and/or negatives in the eccentric phase will maximize size gains for athletes interested in developing muscle bulk.

When doing negative and forced rep sets, the amount of stress the muscles are exposed to is very high. You have to limit the total number of sets and make sure adequate time is allowed between these types of workouts before doing them again.

Workouts incorporating forced reps or negatives should be performed no more than your recuperative abilities will allow. For recreational athletes this may mean one to two times per month for each muscle group. For the elite athlete these sets may be performed as frequently as once a week. It is also best to limit either negative or forced reps to the final one or two sets for any given body part.

Speed Is the Key

The speed you perform the concentric phase of each contraction will determine whether you obtain benefits in muscle strength or power. Concentric muscle contractions performed in a slow, controlled fashion develop muscle strength. Performing them fast and explosively develops muscle power. Because you will be performing the movements quickly, you'll see that the weights you are using are relatively light (20 to 40 percent of your 1RM). Strength training involving slow contractions will result in negligible increases in muscle power, but will allow all the muscle fibers to be trained and will give the muscle tone without adding bulk or size. To develop muscle size, use eccentric contractions. By the nature of the movement, they must be performed slowly.

However, power and size training pose higher risks of injury due to their type of contraction or speed and the additional stress it places on the body. Because of this, you must develop adequate muscle strength with slow-velocity training prior to beginning either power or size training. As with all training, proper form and adequate recovery are critical if adaptations are to take place without setbacks or injuries.

TRAINING GOAL	SPEED OF MOVEMENT	TYPE OF CONTRACTION
Strength	slow-velocity	focus on concentric phase
Power	fast-velocity	focus on concentric phase
Size	slow-velocity	focus on eccentric phase (negatives / forced reps)

You can see that the speed with which you perform a lift and the type of contraction you're focusing on will determine the adaptation that will take place. Using the set and repetition guidelines, athletes can gear their workouts accordingly.

12

GOING THE DISTANCE:
TRAINING FOR ENDURANCE

Whether you are training to improve your performance in a 10K run, century bicycle ride, tennis, or soccer or basketball, you require a certain amount of endurance in order to excel at your game. Endurance is classically defined as the ability to maintain an activity for a prolonged period of time. Therefore, it is a key component of many competitive sports.

Training to maximize your endurance capacity will allow you to improve and enhance your performance in all sports requiring cardiovascular fitness. The guidelines for cardiovascular conditioning given by the ACSM to perform aerobic exercise 3 to 5 days per week for 20 to 60 minutes at an exercise intensity of 65 to 90 percent of your HRmax develop a base level of fitness that allows you to participate in games and sports on a recreational level. For competition, you need a higher fitness level and a more focused and advanced training and conditioning program.

The Short and Long of Intervals

Although endurance is usually thought of in terms of aerobic activities and cardiovascular fitness, your muscles also come into play. If they do not have the necessary adaptations, the heart will deliver oxygen to the muscles, but they won't be sufficiently trained to process it.

To train the muscles and improve their aerobic capacity, you are going to need high-intensity intervals. Continuous training—steadily paced exercise performed at 65 to 75% of your HRmax—is an excellent way to improve cardiovascular health and to get a fitness base in the specific muscles that you use in the activity. But, as the saying goes, these long, slow, distance workouts (LSD) make you great at long, slow distance. With LSD training alone, when the pace goes up in competition, the athlete often begins to suffer. To improve performance and heighten fitness levels, interval training, which places additional stress on your body, is just what the doctor ordered.

There are two main types of intervals: aerobic, or long intervals, which involve training at or, preferably, slightly above your race pace; and anaerobic, or short, intervals, which require you to train well above your race pace and sometimes above your maximal aerobic capacity. Whether long or short, these segments are always performed at intensities above your race pace. The accumulation of lactic acid in the muscles and blood causes a fairly rapid onset of fatigue.

Intervals thus not only include a number of high-intensity segments, but also recovery periods performed for specified periods of time at a comfortable intensity. Recovery is important because it allows you to restore some of your energy stores and remove the lactic acid that has built up during the work interval so that you complete the workout.

The on-time for intervals varies with short intervals performed for 30 to 90 second intervals and long intervals for 3 to 5 minutes. The duration of recovery intervals vary, with work to rest (W:R) ratios ranging from 2:1 or 1:1 for long intervals all the way to 1:3 or 1:4 for short intervals. At times the W:R ratio is more of an art than a science. What is most important is to allow an adequate recovery time between work intervals so that your heart rate returns to normal and exercise intensity can be maintained for subsequent intervals. If your intensity (as measured by speed, pace, etc.) begins to drop, either the recovery interval needs to be lengthened or it is an indication that your body is tired and done with that workout.

Even though the total on-time for intervals is from 5 to 25 minutes, each interval workout should last an hour or more, since you also need to include an adequate warm-up, the time for the recovery intervals, and an adequate cooldown that should include flexibility training.

This high-intensity exercise workout recruits the fast twitch muscle fibers and trains their metabolic systems to become more aerobic and less anaerobic. They therefore produce less lactic acid in subsequent workouts, delaying the onset of fatigue. Although intervals are more difficult to perform, they will help you reach a higher anaerobic threshold and be able to work at an increasingly intense pace for longer periods of time with an increased ability to tolerate higher levels of lactic acid.

Science Matters: Lactate Acid Thresholds

Increasing your lactate threshold is dependent on high intensity, anaerobic interval conditioning. This is in direct contrast to low-to-moderate intensity workouts. During these continuous workouts, ATP energy production only produces smaller, more manageable amounts of lactic acid, which are easily oxidized (or used for energy).

These physiological and biochemical changes in your body's muscle cells improve the cells' ability to generate ATP aerobically, even at higher exercise intensities. This in turn lets you participate at a higher percentage of your VO_2max for a longer time than you would have been able to before.

Lactic acid begins to accumulate and rise quickly at about 50 to 55 percent of an untrained person's maximal aerobic capacity (VO_2max), but if you are highly conditioned, it can occur at 80 to 90 percent of your VO_2max. At some point, however, you will reach your anaerobic threshold (more precisely called your blood lactate threshold), and will be unable to perform at intensities above it for prolonged periods of time. Your race pace, or maximum steady state (MSS), is just below this threshold.

Rather than going to a lab to find out precisely what their VO_2max or lactate threshold is, most athletes use their heart rate at their race pace as a measurement for training intensities. While portable lactate monitors are available, heart rate is a much easier and acceptable means of gauging training intensity.

Because interval training involves working out at levels that are more intense than normal, the risk of injury associated with it is greater. In addition, these intensity levels and the increased buildup of lactic acid will make the workouts more demanding and, at times, uncomfortable. For these reasons, it is best not to participate in structured interval training until an adequate fitness base is developed. A base usually takes two to three months.

You may, however, make use of a less demanding technique called Fartlek training. Unlike more structured intervals, Fartlek training has you vary the intensity at will. Because these intervals are not as structured, they are less intense than standard intervals. They will, however, be at intensities higher than the levels you are normally accustomed to and will impart at least some of the benefits of interval training.

In early parts of the training season, high-intensity workouts make up a small percentage of your total training, with interval training being done at most once every two weeks. The bulk of this base training phase is composed of long duration, low-to-moderate intensity continuous training. As your fitness levels improve, high-intensity interval workouts are increased to at most once or twice a week. To allow for adaptations and recovery, these workouts must be interspersed with easy-to-moderate recovery workouts. Often, one long duration workout per week is added, so you can gradually work up to the amount of time you will spend in the event or competition.

Athletes not involved in traditional aerobic sports often use their sports for their cardiovascular conditioning rather than long, steady runs or rides and perform one to two days per week of intervals on the track, road, or field to raise their overall performance.

Below is a summary table describing the different types of intervals as well as features of each.

INTERVAL TYPE	INTERVAL DURATION	W : R RATIO	INTERVAL INTENSITY	INTERVAL EXAMPLE	PRIMARY BENEFITS
Short/ Anaerobic	30 to 90 seconds	1:1 to 1:4	> VO_2max	400m run 1k bike	speed efficiency
Long/ Aerobic	3 to 5 minutes	2:1 to 1:1	> MSS	mile run 3k bike	sustained power

For the entire interval you will exercise at the highest intensity that allows you to complete the duration at maximal effort. Athletes involved in endurance events or sports lasting at least 60 minutes perform more aerobic intervals to develop a high degree of sustained speed, while anaerobic intervals are done by athletes whose events last less than an hour and who require a high amount of explosive speed (or power) along with endurance.

VO_2max and Performance

Maximal aerobic capacity (VO_2max) measures the maximal amount of oxygen per unit of time that the body can process while exercising. VO_2max is an indication of your body's capacity to utilize oxygen and perform aerobic exercise and is commonly used to denote an individual's fitness. For the general public, the higher an individual's VO_2max, the better they'll perform in endurance activities.

VO_2max is a function of oxygen delivery and oxygen utilization. To improve oxygen delivery, the cardiovascular systems must be trained and its function enhanced. Improving oxygen utilization during exercise enhances the aerobic capacity of the muscle involved in the sport.

The intensity of training that improves the function of the cardiovascular system is not the same intensity of training that improves the muscular system. Continuous, long steady distance training at low-to-moderate intensities will improve oxygen delivery, cardiovascular function, and overall cardiovascular fitness. High-intensity interval training increases the muscle's oxygen utilization capacity, which will improve overall performance because higher intensities can be maintained for longer periods of time.

VO_2max is a good but not flawless indicator of elite performance because it does not guarantee how efficient the utilization system is. The table below shows hypothetical physiological data on two athletes. It relates VO_2max and the maximal steady state (MSS) for exercise performance as indicated by marathon times.

	VO₂MAX	MSS, RELATIVE	MSS, ABSOLUTE	MARATHON TIME
Athlete One	87 ml/kg/min	75 percent VO_2max	65.25 ml/kg/min	2:16:00
Athlete Two	80 ml/kg/min	85 percent VO_2max	68 ml/kg/min	2:10:00

The equation used to calculate marathon time is: running speed = (VO_2max − 3.5) / 0.2

As shown in the table, although athlete one has a higher VO_2max, the differences in their maximal steady states permits athlete two to perform at a higher intensity and run a faster marathon, assuming all other factors are equal. This is because the race pace is equivalent to running at one's steady-state threshold, not one's VO_2max. While VO_2max is an indicator of performance exercise, this intensity can't be maintained for long without exhaustion due to the buildup of lactic acid. Unlike exercise at VO_2max, exercise at an intensity equivalent to steady state can. Therefore, knowing your steady-state threshold, and more important knowing how to adapt (raise) it, is actually a better predictor of endurance performance than VO_2max.

Because MSS is dependent upon the aerobic capacity of fast-twitch fibers, higher intensity training must be incorporated into your workouts to recruit, utilize and condition the fast-twitch fibers. Fast-twitch muscle fibers with higher aerobic capacities allow individuals to exercise at higher intensities before utilizing anaerobic pathways. This results in less lactic acid buildup and a later onset of fatigue.

Muscle Fiber Types

Muscles are composed of two fiber types: slow twitch and fast twitch. Slow-twitch fibers are used for posture and primarily for aerobic, low-intensity exercise. Fast-twitch fibers, which are responsible for explosive power and help give the muscle its tone, are called into play at high-intensity activities, which are often anaerobic.

Low-to-moderate intensity workouts, therefore, primarily recruit slow-twitch muscle fibers. As exercise intensity increases, your muscles start to use the fast-twitch fibers as well. It is not until maximal force is required that all the fibers are called into play.

Studies on the muscle-fiber composition of athletes have found endurance athletes to have higher percentages of slow-twitch muscle fibers (up to 90 percent in the leg muscles of runners) and power athletes to have a higher percentage of fast-twitch muscle fibers (80 percent fast twitch in the leg muscles of sprinters). Fast-twitch muscle fibers generate more force more quickly than slow-twitch muscle fibers, which is why people with more fast-twitch muscle fibers do better at high-intensity activities. Unlike elite athletes with muscle composed of primarily one fiber type, most individuals are born with a mixture of fiber types with a fairly even distribution of fast- and slow-twitch muscle fibers (50 percent fast and 50 percent slow). While exercise training can alter the metabolic properties of a muscle fiber (improving the aerobic or anaerobic capacity), training does little to change a muscle fiber's contractile property. We are born with a specific muscle fiber distribution. And because muscle fiber types are one of the prime factors in predicting an individual's performance potential, Olympic endurance athletes are born as much as they are bred.

While slow-twitch fibers are used at all exercise intensities, they perform relatively little work at high exercise intensities because the fast-twitch fibers generate the most force. However, one of the metabolic by-products of fast-twitch fibers and high-intensity training is a temporary buildup of lactic acid in the muscles. As fast-twitch fibers become more accustomed to the demands of high-intensity aerobic training, they produce lower amounts of lactic acid and have an increased aerobic capacity. In addition, the whole body adapts by being better able to handle high lactate levels.

Calculating Your Training Zones

Using your heart rate to measure exercise intensity while training for endurance is excellent for feedback and accuracy. Both percentage of heart rate max (HRmax), as described earlier, and percentage of heart rate reserve (HRR) are used in research and in practical settings.

While using one's percent of HRmax to calculate exercise intensity is easy and effective for the general fitness enthusiast, using a percentage of one's heart rate reserve (HRR) is more accurate for elite athletes. This is because the Karvonen formula used to determine %HRR takes into account one's fitness level, using resting heart rate (RHR) in the equation, and as you get fitter your resting heart rate drops. It is not uncommon for elite, endurance athletes to have a resting heart rate ranging from 30 to 40 beats per minute while the average person's RHR is 70 to 75 beats per minute. The heart of the trained individual is stronger and can therefore beat harder and pump more blood with each beat.

There is also a more direct relationship between the percentage of HRR and the percentage of VO_2max that gives a more accurate setting of exercise intensity and also takes into account one's fitness level. To calculate the appropriate exercise intensity the equation used is the Karvonen formula, which is calculated as:

$$[(220 - age) - RHR) \times \text{Training Percentage}] + RHR$$

The recommended training zone for continuous workouts is between 50 and 85 percent of HRR based on the Karvonen formula. Below is an example of how to calculate the training sensitive zone based on percent HRR utilizing the Karvonen formula.

CONDITION	AGE	RHR	LOW END OF ZONE (50% HRR)	HIGH END OF ZONE (85% HRR)
Unfit subject	20 years	70 bpm	$[(220 - 20) - 70) \times 0.5]$ + 70 = **135 bpm**	$[(220 - 20) - 70) \times 0.85]$ + 70 = **181 bpm**
Fit subject	20 years	35 bpm	$[(220 - 20) - 35) \times 0.5]$ + 35 = **118 bpm**	$[(220 - 20) - 35) \times 0.85]$ + 35 = **175 bpm**

For convenience, most people count their heartbeats for 10 seconds and then multiply by six to get the heart beats per minute. They then compare their working heart rate with the desired number calculated using the above equation. For true convenience, some people wear heart rate monitors, which do all of the math for you.

It is also important to note that using the equation of (220 − age) to calculate the age-predicted maximal heart rate (HRmax) to determine your training zone has its limitations. There is a margin of error of +/− 12 to 15 beats per minute. For masters athletes who have been active their entire life, the equation often under predicts their maximal heart rate capacity and therefore under predicts their optimal training zone. With this in mind, athletes will often use the highest heart rate they can achieve during a maximal workout as their HRmax for calculation purposes.

Rating of Perceived Exertion (RPE)

Without the use of a heart-rate monitor, having to measure exercise heart rate by hand during a workout can become cumbersome and distracting. While exercise heart rate is essential for intervals, knowing your precise workout heart rate is not as critical for other workouts.

Athletes often go by how they feel during a particular workout to gauge their training intensity. The Rating of Perceived Exertion (RPE) is an easier, practical way to monitor the workout's intensity. Because experienced athletes tend to estimate the extent of their efforts correctly, RPE is their monitoring method of choice for continuous workouts.

RPE uses research done in the mid-1980s by scientists such as Gunnar Borg, who developed a scale correlating perception with the actual effort. In the newest, revised version of the scale, which goes from a value of 1 (nothing at all) to 10 (very, very strong), the training sensitive zone based on HRR of 50 to 85 percent corresponds to an RPE of 3 to 7, which classifies the exercise intensity as moderate (3) to severe (7). If you are a 20-year-old whose low-end training zone is 135 beats per minute, the effort that you perceived at a heart rate of 135 corresponds to a 3 on the RPE scale. As your fitness level increases, the intensity with which you can maintain continuous activity will also increase. You will thus have a similar RPE, but will be at a greater exercise intensity.

If you haven't used RPE before, pay attention to your breathing patterns. If you are gasping for breath and can't talk through a complete sentence, you are probably in the eight to nine range. If you have extreme breathlessness, you've exceeded your anaerobic threshold. Muscle burn and severe discomfort are also indications that you are above your zone.

Avoiding Burnout

Balancing training and recovery to match fitness levels is a key to avoiding signs and symptoms of overtraining. The overtraining symptoms may persist for days, weeks, or even months depending on the severity and until the athlete gets adequate rest.

Nutritional factors play a key role in the recovery process, with carbohydrates being the most important. High-intensity workouts gradually deplete muscle and liver glycogen levels. Resupplying the body's carbohydrate stores takes time, even if you're on a diet high in carbohydrates. Reduced training or complete rest, combined with a high carbohydrate intake (up to 10 grams per kilogram of body weight) is necessary to reestablish pre-exercise glycogen levels after high-intensity, exhaustive training or competition.

Too Much of a Good Thing: Overtraining

Very few of us factor the demands of the recovery period into our training schedules. Instead, we think of training simply as the workout, or period of daily exercise. We don't think about recovery, and wonder why our workouts have become more painful or more boring.

How do you know if you are overtrained? Overtraining is measured as a drop in physical performance associated with lethargy, decreased motivation, generalized fatigue, and a compromised immune system. It is an indication that the training stress is in excess of the body's ability to adapt and recover. And, as any sports medicine doctor or psychologist can tell you, it's an epidemic.

An unexpected side effect of the fitness boom is the modern phenomenon of the "sick" athlete. While many of us have taken the prescription to exercise to heart, we haven't been as good with our diet or with restraint. Particularly during the early stages of a rigorous training program and just before a competitive event, we force an unrelentingly intense amount of stress on our bodies. Unless our diet and recovery time compensate for that stress, we encourage depleted nutrient stores, overtraining injuries, low-grade viral infections, and muscle soreness. They are natural responses to a body that has been pushed beyond reason.

It is not surprising athletes behave this way: The same motivation that gives someone the discipline to train and win is the same motivation that makes us particularly prone to push ourselves to the max. This is compounded by the demand in society in general for immediate results. Both as athletes and as professionals, we have been taught to mistrust the concept of rest, and treat it—as well as patience—as a sign of weakness.

Furthermore, despite warnings to the contrary, many of us still live our lives under the "no pain, no gain" motto. Because we are programmed for action, we accept soreness and fatigue as badges of honor—if it hurts, it must be working. So rather than take time off to let our bodies adapt, we all too often push ourselves through another workout thinking that we're doing our bodies a favor.

We're not. We may think we're training for optimal performance, but we're really overtraining. And that can be dangerous.

There are several ways scientists can measure the amount of stress exercise places on the body, including blood and urine tests and monitoring weight changes, motivation and decreases in performance. But there is one simple test for overtraining that you can do yourself. It involves measuring your resting heart rate each morning.

Start by taking and recording your morning pulse first thing upon waking for seven to ten days. To take your pulse, lie quietly and place your index and middle finger of one hand on your opposite wrist, toward the thumb side. Once you feel your pulse, count each beat for 60 seconds. That will give you your resting heart rate at that time. If possible, do this during a period when the stress level in your life is at a minimal or at least manageable level.

Once you've got the figures, average them together to get your average resting pulse. Use this as your baseline. An elevation of as little as 10 percent indicates stress, be it physical or psychological, from your training, illness, injury, personal or professional life. A 20 percent increase, especially for more than two days, is a red flag that you may be overtrained. If you continue to train hard, you will be.

Remember: Exercise is not the only stress in your life. Other stressors in your life will limit your ability to respond positively to the additional stress of training. If you are really emotionally stressed out, rest, recovery, and nutrition are more critical in maintaining your health and progress than exercise.

To avoid putting yourself at greater risk, pay special attention to your diet. If your resting pulse is elevated by more than 10 percent, reduce the intensity and/or duration of your training on that day. If it's elevated by more than 20 percent, take a rest day.

All Pain Is Not Created Equal

A second factor that may indicate or predict whether you are overtrained has to do with pain. Pain can range from mild discomfort to debilitating agony, and can be brought about by stimulation of specialized nerve endings that alert the brain to the fact that something damaging has or is about to occur. Because there is a world of difference between the pain caused by an overuse injury and the soreness that follows a difficult workout, you should learn how to distinguish between the types of pain you might feel during or after a workout.

One type of pain, characterized by postponed soreness, is symptomatic of a normal response called delayed onset muscle soreness

(DOMS). It rarely begins during the workout. More often, it appears several hours after a workout, and peaks about 24 hours later. Typically, the pain disappears within five to seven days.

This soreness usually isn't indicative of any real problem, so you should continue training, albeit at a reduced intensity. Lighter activity helps the repair process by increasing blood flow to the area. This in turn removes waste products, increases metabolism, and helps supply required nutrients to the sore muscles.

Overuse Injuries

Overuse injuries are a much different story. They are painful not just after, but during the workout. Because they are the result of overtraining or of cumulative stress on the body, they don't peak a day later. Instead, they usually get worse and often become chronic conditions. As anyone who has lived with chronic pain can tell you, this pain is not something that you can ignore. Ultimately, it interferes with your ability to enjoy life.

One of the most common overuse injuries among athletes is connective tissue damage within the muscle, tendon, ligament, or cartilage of our joints. The cartilage in joints such as the knee or shoulder is vulnerable to a wide range of traumas. When a joint becomes inflamed, the body can't supply as much blood to the joint. Without this blood, the body can't easily repair the cartilage or the ligaments in the joint. Over time, the degeneration in cartilage can lead to chronic aches and pains, osteoarthritis, and immobility.

The problem intensifies as we get older because aging destroys our natural antioxidant enzyme systems. Under optimal conditions,

The Overtraining Checklist

One of the most common causes of illness or injury in athletes comes from overuse. Being overtrained is more than a short-term dip in competitive level performance or inability to train as hard as usual. Training too much or too hard for one's fitness level often results in overtraining signs and symptoms including:

- An unexplained drop in performance.
- Psychological disturbances including depression, generalized fatigue, and irritability.
- Physiological disturbances including GI tract disturbances, elevated resting heart rate, and hormonal disturbances indicative of stress.
- Sleep disturbances and insomnia.
- Decrease in appetite and weight loss.
- Increased susceptibility to upper respiratory tract infections and colds. Persistent flulike symptoms. A cold that just won't go away.
- Increased incidence of training specific overuse injuries to muscles and connective tissues.
- A loss of interest in training.
- Excessive muscle soreness and muscle weakness.
- A prolonged increase in resting heart rate (by 10% or more).

our bodies have innate defenses against free radicals, which damage cell components and impair proper function. Without effective levels of natural antioxidants as a line of defense, the connective tissue is vulnerable to these free radicals, which can trigger a further degeneration of connective tissue structure and function.

The onset of connective tissue damage can be subtle. Stiffness could be the first symptom, followed by pain when you move the joint. Because these injuries are the result of cumulative stress, they logically worsen as we get older or increase our training intensity. Not so long ago, we probably would have accepted these conditions as natural consequences of the aging process. Now we can take a more positive approach to an overuse injury, regardless of our age.

These overtraining-related injuries are in fact the most common form of injury that plague recreational and elite athletes. In the past, most of us would have tried to push through the pain. But now we know that this only elevates your risk of joint and muscle injuries, leaves you vulnerable to low-level infections, aches and pains, and compromises your immune system.

The best way to both prevent and treat these injuries is to give the muscles sufficient time to recover, to provide the body with the depleted nutrients, and to supply the body with adequate additional nutrients for growth and adaptation.

PART IV

SPECIAL CONSIDERATIONS

13

SPECIAL CONSIDERATIONS FOR THE YOUNG ATHLETE

Just as children involved in sports must be provided with proper equipment and supervision because of the risk of injury inherent in any physical activity, children must also be provided with the best possible diet. Particular attention needs to be paid to children in weight-dependent sports, who are often vulnerable to eating disorders and a variety of health-related consequences such as premature loss of bone mass.

Do They Need More?

The balance of energy nutrients for children past the age of two and adolescents is similar to that of adults. Only infants have been shown to require higher amounts of fat and cholesterol in their diets than others. Children need more micronutrients on a per kilogram body weight basis than adolescents and adults, but by age eleven many levels are similar to adult values. A balanced and healthy diet

157

will supply most of these nutrients in adequate amounts, particularly with the fortification found in many cereals, sports drinks, and foods.

Vital Water

In terms of nutrient intakes, water is vitally important because compared to adults, children produce more heat relative to body mass during exercise, have lower sweat rates, and greater rises in their core temperatures with dehydration. For this reason, regular drinking in volumes greater than dictated by thirst alone must be encouraged and implemented as part of training.

Introducing water early in development, as early as one year, will develop a child's taste for it. As long as your child is getting adequate nutrition and calories, diluting juice one-to-one with water can be a helpful first step and will reduce the caloric density. Many juices, particularly apple juice, have a high sugar content and contain few additional nutrients, making them only slightly better than soda. One hundred percent orange juice and grapefruit juice with pulp not only provide more micronutrients, but also add some fiber to the drink, making them superior food choices. (They are not good for our teeth in large and frequent amounts, though. The acid in them tends to break down tooth enamel.)

It almost goes without saying that the most effective way to get your child to drink an adequate amount of water is by setting a good example yourself. Choose water over a soda, coffee, or other beverages. It will benefit both you and your child.

Weighty Matters

For children with weight problems, activity is the primary key to weight loss and lifelong weight management. Youths who are inactive need to be more active, not eat less. However, wise food choices are also vital. Switching from a diet high in fat, calorically dense, and rich in processed foods to one which is primarily plant based and low in fat provides them with essential nutrients without excessive calories.

Repeatedly, studies on both boys and girls have shown that, like adults, obese and overweight children eat significantly fewer calories than children of normal weight. They are also significantly less active both in terms of exercise and spontaneous movement throughout the day. For example, time-in-motion photographic studies showed that obese children spent four hours in physical activity and normal weight children spent eleven hours per week.

This pattern begins very early in life. Infants of obese parents tend to have significantly lower metabolisms and less spontaneous activities in their cribs than infants of normal-weight parents. Genetics can play a role in the development of obesity, but obesity appears to be controllable through diet and lifestyle modification.

It takes six to eight weeks to modify eating habits and food and taste preferences, many of which were learned early in life. So start slowly. In a short time you should be able to significantly reduce the amount of salt, processed sweets, and fat from your child's diet. Within months they'll be able to go from whole fat to low fat and eventually nonfat dairy products. Soon low-fat milk, which at first tasted like gray water to them, will seem too heavy. The desire for salty foods will also diminish as you limit the amount found in the foods they eat, particularly the processed ones.

Television: The Hidden Culprit

Childhood obesity is also linked to television. Astonishingly, two-thirds of all kids up to age eighteen and one-quarter of two- to four-year-olds have television sets in their bedrooms. In addition, the average child watches twenty-four hours of television each week. This is disturbing for numerous reasons, not the least of which is the link between TV and childhood obesity.

A study at Harvard Medical School found that the likelihood of obesity is linked to the number of hours young children and teenagers watch TV. The study found that the prevalence of obesity increased 2 percent for every hour of television they watched per day. The younger TV watching begins, the heavier children tend to be.

It is not just that TV encourages kids to be less active, but that it constantly reinforces bad food choices. Many programs and ads typically encourage a desire for high-calorie snacks, sweets, and overly refined foods.

As a result, limiting sedentary time watching television or playing video or computer games to less than ten hours a week is a good idea and a significant reduction from the twenty-four-hour average of today's kids.

Food cues also play into the emotional void many of these children have and teach them to eat when they are bored, stressed out, or feeling unloved. That is why you should not feed your child's emotional hunger with food. Rather than use food as a reward or as a substitute for nurturing, meet their emotional needs with time, love, and family activities. That doesn't mean you should forbid them from eating their favorite foods altogether, because that will merely make these foods more attractive. Just make sure that they only eat them occasionally, and that they always have an array of healthier foods available to them.

Supplements—Is There a Substitute?

Few, if any, studies have been performed looking at the short- or long-term safety of supplementation by children or adolescents. At this age, optimal training, nutrition, and recovery are far more important than a reliance on supplements for sports enhancement: Teaching them to rely on the latest "magic potion" is counterproductive. As with your diet, supplements for your child should be added as protection, not a substitute for a healthy diet. A daily one-a-day vitamin and mineral supplement is all they'll need, active or not.

Activity, Not Training

Physical activity as play is very important for all kids—big and small. Exercise establishes a metabolism that is efficient at burning foods rather than storing them. It influences the hormones and enzymes working in kids' cells and the level of nutrients in their bloodstream. Exercise also increases the amount of muscle in children's bodies, increases their bone density, and decreases body fat levels. So besides helping to develop a healthy body, you will be developing healthy lifestyle choices that pay off not only today but for their lifetimes.

Too much, just like too little, exercise may have adverse effects on development. A good goal is to have your child be vigorously active for at least one to preferably two hours a day. It doesn't have to be all at once. The activity is best when it is play and not "training." Encourage activities such as dancing, rollerblading, riding a bike, swimming, running, or tag, as well as anything their imagination comes up with. As long as they are moving, their bodies are benefiting from activity. By keeping this play unstructured, you'll reinforce the joy of activity and reduce the chance they'll burn out on sports by the time they grow up.

14

THE FEMALE ATHLETE

Many female athletes are concerned not only with their performance, but also with the cultural pressure to be thin. Because they may be afraid to gain weight, they are more likely than their male counterparts to skip meals, skimp on calories, or eat poorly. Although the dietary habits of athletes vary widely from individual to individual and sport to sport, several studies of athletes from the high school level to Olympic caliber consistently indicate that females tend to have more nutrient deficiencies than males of a similar ability level.

Part of this is due to their overall lower caloric intake. Inadequate caloric intake often inhibits recovery and leads to overtraining, injury, and burnout. Without adequate calories, carbohydrates, and proteins, the body cannot recover from intense workouts. Several studies have found that the level of carbohydrates in the diets of female athletes are below those recommended for endurance athletes. When carbohydrates are in short supply, muscle glycogen stores become depleted, which will compromise both muscle power and endurance.

Female athletes from a wide variety of sports also have inadequate protein intakes for their activity levels. Limited protein intake can lead to inadequate repair of vital components within the muscle cells and slow the repair needed from the workouts. The athletic groups most susceptible to inadequate calorie and nutrient intakes include ballet dancers, basketball players, bodybuilders, gymnasts, runners, skiers, swimmers, triathletes, and wrestlers, because these athletes are more likely to be attempting to control or lose weight.

Most of the studies on female athletes and micronutrient intake have found significant nutrient deficiencies in iron, zinc, calcium, and several of the B vitamins. Most of these studies were surveys that compared nutrient intakes relative to a standard, such as the RDA, and have not analyzed performance capacity or the effects that the dietary deficiency had on athletic performance. Since the RDA or other standards incorporate a safety margin, it may be possible that the athlete will not develop a nutrient deficiency. Even if the athlete does not develop a true nutrient deficiency, her athletic performance may deteriorate and her risk of exercise-related injuries may increase.

The Female Athlete Triad

It is not just athletic performance that may suffer. Restrictive diets and eating disorders in female athletes may contribute to the development of premature osteoporosis. This has prompted the ACSM to develop a position on the Female Athlete Triad; a combination of disordered eating, amenorrhea (absence or irregular stoppage of menses), and osteoporosis. Although the exact cause has not been identified, the underlying behavior leading to these problems appears to be disordered eating. Females who don't take in enough calories in order to improve their appearance and/or competitive ability in sports probably are not meeting their energy and protein needs. They may also be exercising excessively to burn calories. This combination of restrictive caloric intake with compulsive exercise affects their hormonal balance and predisposes them to irregular menstrual patterns and osteoporosis.

Calcium and Your Bones

One major health benefit of exercise for females is that weight-bearing exercise has proven to be beneficial in increasing bone density. The mechanical stress of exercise facilitates bone development and the deposition of calcium into bone. This, however, is true only for weight-bearing exercise like running, volleyball, gymnastics, weight lifting, and other impact-sport activities, but not the case for nonimpact sports like swimming, whose participants often have bone densities below that of sedentary females. Results from one recent study suggest that exercise can be used to help maintain and increase bone mineral density in postmenopausal females. It is important to note that only those bones that are stressed during the activity are affected.

A recent survey of women found that one of the nutrients that they are often deficient in is calcium, particularly in the early developmental years. This deficient intake, especially when combined with high-protein diets, increases the risk of osteoporosis later in life. While exercise will be beneficial at maintaining bone densities, eating a diet high in calcium, with adequate but not excessive protein, is extremely important for bone development, particularly throughout the first three decades of life when bone density can increase. After this point, bone density is steadily lost as one continues to age. To maximize bone density, all females, especially if they are athletic, should be sure to take in the recommended dose of calcium: 1,200 milligrams per day. While calcium is absorbed best from natural sources such as nonfat dairy products, supplements can be used as well.

Iron—Essential for Women

Iron is a micronutrient of particular concern for the female athlete, particularly when she is premenopausal and losing iron-rich blood as a result of menstruation. A second concern is a type of anemia called "runner's anemia." Red blood cell damage, increased losses through perspiration, and an increased blood volume in athletes may account for the additional iron losses seen in athletes, particularly runners. Adolescent and adult premenopausal females require more dietary iron, 15 milligrams per day, than males' 10 to 12 milligrams per day.

While decreased iron stores and hemoglobin levels can reduce athletic performance, random supplementation is not recommended due to the possibility of toxicity. Female runners and other athletes can regularly have their hemoglobin and iron status measured to determine the need for increased dietary intakes of iron or the need for supplementation. Females, especially endurance athletes, must include iron-rich foods in their diet or risk incurring iron-deficiency anemia and impaired athletic performance. If you are taking an iron supplement, it is best to take it with citrus juice because vitamin C increases its absorption. Do not, however, take it with milk or other dairy products or tea because these decrease iron bioavailability.

Menstruation and the Female Athlete

Premenstrual syndrome is a disorder found in some women a few days prior to menstruation. Common symptoms include depression, anxiety, bloating, headache, and mood swings. While vitamin B6 is commonly used to treat PMS symptoms, toxic side effects of excessive megadose amounts of vitamin B6, such as permanent nerve damage, numbness in the hands and feet, and difficulties walking are common.

While the cause of PMS is unclear, eating a balanced diet while limiting caffeine, alcohol, nicotine, and salt may reduce its symptoms. Several herbal remedies have been found to be beneficial including chasteberry, black cohosh, and evening primrose oil. Several are used by European and English doctors for the treatment of PMS symptoms. In the U.S., on the other hand, we often prescribe the hormone progesterone, even though it has as little as a 50 percent success rate.

Amenorrhea (absence or irregular stoppage of menses) is much more common among female athletes than their sedentary counterparts. As many as 30 percent of all competitive runners, gymnasts, and bodybuilders are amenorrheic, which has a negative impact on

Don't Sweat It

As most of you are aware, there is a distinct difference in the amount of sweat produced by men and women. Although women possess more sweat glands than men, they generally sweat less. It appears that most women rely more on circulatory mechanisms to dissipate heat, whereas most men rely more on evaporative cooling. Those individuals who sweat even more need to be extremely conscious of their overall fluid intake during and after exercise.

Menstruation does play a role in a female's response to exercise. Women sweat less during the two weeks prior to the onset of menstruation and sweat more during the two weeks following the onset of menstruation. While this change in temperature regulation does not affect a woman's athletic performance, it will change her fluid requirements during different parts of her menstrual cycle.

their bones. Due to the drop in their estrogen levels, they lose the premenopausal protective effect of estrogens on maintenance of bone density and suffer more exercise-induced stress fractures. Several studies have found the bone densities of amenorrheic runners to be below those of sedentary, normally menstruating females, and even further below runners with normal menstrual cycles.

Exercise does not counteract the negative consequences of amenorrhea. Reducing the training overload, increasing caloric intake, and modifying stress levels are all beneficial for returning the female athlete to her normal menstrual pattern and reducing the negative health consequences of amenorrhea.

The Pregnant Athlete

The American College of Obstetrics and Gynecology now suggests all women participate in a regular exercise program during pregnancy, for the health of both the mother and the fetus. Besides the additional calories and protein required for activity and exercise, pregnancy demands additional nutrient intakes. For a healthy weight gain of 25 to 35 pounds, an average pregnant female requires approximately 300 additional calories per day during the second and third trimesters. No additional caloric intake is needed during the first trimester. Note that this amount is not equivalent to twice the normal caloric intake, even though the mother is now "eating for two."

To avoid dehydration and overheating, pregnant women must also drink plenty of fluids, particularly during and after exercise. In addition, pregnant women need an additional 15 grams of protein, 5 micrograms of vitamin D, 220 micrograms of folic acid, 400 mg calcium, 15 mg iron, 40 mg magnesium, and three mg zinc. With the exception of iron, these can all be obtained through food. Iron is the only supplement that the National Academy of Sciences recommends during pregnancy. However, most physicians prescribe a prenatal multi-vitamin and mineral supplement along with a separate iron supplement for protection.

As Strong As Men?

Who cares? In the past 20 years, women have broken virtually every athletic barrier that had been placed in their way. As they make their way into professional and semi-professional sports, performance is every bit as important to them as it is to men. Other than the issues covered in this chapter, their concerns are the same as men's and vary only in terms of their body weight. In fact, studies have shown that they are also more vigilant about their training and diet. That, even more than strength, is the mark of a real competitor.

15

GETTING BACK ON TRACK

The last thing you want to be is injured or sick. Unfortunately, from time to time, you are bound to be one or the other. Most athletes are familiar with the RICE prescription (rest, ice, compression, and elevation), which works for minor injuries. There are, however, several nutritional options beyond chicken soup you can use to speed the healing and recovery process. Because there is limited research to support these claims, many physicians will not know or recommend these nutrients. But they often are surprised by the results.

Does Nutrition Work?

Jason, a fifty-year-old publishing executive, completely shattered and crushed the bones and tendons in his ankle in a car crash. He knew he had months, if not years, of therapy to come following his multiple surgeries. In fact, his doctors gave him little hope of ever regaining function in the joint and felt he was lucky they had been able to save his foot.

Having had personal experience with trauma injuries and the literature surrounding them, I recommended that Jason take additional protein, vitamins, minerals, and glucosamine sulfate to speed his recovery from reconstructive ankle surgery. Like most physicians, Jason's orthopedic specialist was skeptical about the value of these supplements. Despite his doctor's skepticism, Jason immediately increased his protein, vitamin C, calcium, magnesium, zinc, and glucosamine sulfate intake.

The process of repair, surgeries, and therapy was slow. But on each visit, his doctor was amazed at Jason's progress. In time, he hesitantly acknowledged that the additional nutrients were indeed enhancing his recovery.

Now, Jason and the doctor both agree that the nutritional assist was a critical factor to his recovery. Combined with grueling physical therapy, it helped him not only regain moderate function in his ankle joint, but also to walk unassisted by crutches or a cane in less than 18 months after his accident and first surgery.

This does not mean you should ignore your physician. Rely on him or her for diagnosis and treatment. But you yourself have the most to gain from a speedy recovery. If for that reason alone, play an active role in your own care. Athletes have different requirements from the sedentary population. To get the best information, you want to consult a specialist in sports nutrition. Look for someone with an advanced degree in nutrition or a related field from an accredited educational institution. If you cannot afford or find one, use the resources at the end of this book to research the information yourself.

Although the Internet is an amazing research tool, the information on the web is not regulated, is often disseminated by special interest groups, and frequently misrepresents the research. The websites listed in the resource section are trustworthy. Others may or may not be.

More Than Chicken Soup

The most common malady athletes fall prey to is an increased incidence of upper respiratory tract infections (URTI). Symptoms include a runny nose, sneezing, sore throat, cough, and fever. While moderate exercise heightens immune function, intense exercise and competition have been shown to blunt the body's immune response, which is its first line of defense against infectious agents. This places a person at increased risk of URTI for up to several weeks following the exercise or event.

Generally, the risk of infection is directly related to performance or overload. Runners with faster times or superior performance, for example, experience more symptoms than slower ones. URTI are also more common in athletes with the most strenuous training programs.

Athletes can protect themselves in a number of ways. The first is by obtaining adequate carbohydrates. Carbohydrates help to maintain muscle and liver glycogen stores and therefore limit the negative effects of intense training, the possibility of overtraining, and generalized fatigue. Maintaining appropriate daily intakes of carbohydrates for one's training level before, during, and after exercise will markedly reduce the training stress. High carbohydrate levels after exercise, combined with reduced training, will enhance recovery.

Vitamin C is a second option. While taking vitamin C at levels above the recommended daily level does not protect the general population against URTI, supplementation protects athletes engaging in heavy exercise. In a study of distance runners, those taking 600 milligrams daily (10 times the RDA) immediately before and for three weeks after an ultra-marathon race experienced fewer symptoms of URTI than those receiving a placebo. Based on this research, increase your intake of vitamin C, which best comes primarily from natural sources in fruits and juices. If you need more than your diet supplies, you can make up the difference with an additional 500 milligram vitamin C tablet a day.

Although less widely known, glutamine also plays an important role in normal immune function. Because the levels of glutamine in the blood decrease following prolonged high-intensity exercise, a glutamine deficiency has been linked to the depressed immune function that results from strenuous exercise. Supplementation with glutamine before, during, and after exercise may compensate for this postexercise decline in glutamine associated with intense training. Taking five grams of glutamine immediately after intense workouts, particularly when you're sick or when you are exposed to people who are sick, will help to maintain blood glutamine levels and immune function.

When you're sick, it's particularly important to pay attention to your water and fluid intake. Added fluids help the body rid itself of toxins and other waste products. Diluted juice with water will not only supply fluids, but will provide additional energy and antioxidants you need to combat illness.

Other factors contributing to a depressed immune system include lack of sleep, overall poor nutrition, weight loss, and mental stress. The event or competition itself may also add stress to the system. As a result, stress management is one of the best things you can do to keep your immune response strong.

Once you have an infection, several over-the-counter supplements including zinc lozenges, echinacea, and elderberry extract have been shown to reduce the duration and severity of symptoms from viral infections, including the common cold.

One common recommendation for training when you have a cold or infection is whether the symptoms are above or below your neck. If your symptoms are limited to your sinuses and nose, train, albeit at a significantly reduced intensity. If you have congestion in your lungs or feel weak or sore, skip your workouts for a day or two. Although it may be difficult to miss a workout or two, you'll be back much sooner than pushing through it and potentially complicating matters.

In Addition to Your Physician

While studies have been done on the incidence of illness, the effect of exercise on the immune system, and the role of nutrition in the treatment or prevention of illness in athletes, very little has been done in regards to nutrition for injury treatment or prevention. Because most injuries in sports are the result of overuse, the body needs to recover before it can be prepared for subsequent workouts. And there's no better way to do that than by combining adequate rest with optimal nutrition.

To accelerate the repair process, you need to raise the intake of a few key nutrients. Protein is critical for tissue repair and this is a good time to add more to your diet. Even if you are sedentary during your convalescence, take in a daily amount of protein equal to that set for a moderate-intensity workout day (1.5 grams per kilogram per day). To carve out the optimal environment for cellular repair, don't eat it all at once. Instead, spread the protein consumption throughout the day.

If your injury involves a fracture, additional vitamin C, calcium, magnesium, phosphorus, and zinc—all essential to bone development—may aid in the repair of the bone. Make sure to keep your intake of phosphorus in balance with your calcium intake. Ingesting phosphorus in levels above that of calcium, as is frequently the case with people who drink a lot of soda, results in an increased excretion of both phosphorus and calcium in the urine.

Before You Head to the Medicine Cabinet

Training through pain has led to a casual dependence on anti-inflammatories. If you take over-the-counter anti-inflammatory pills daily, as if they're vitamins, you're like 50 million other Americans, athletes and not.

Anti-inflammatories are big business. Americans alone spend over $2.7 billion dollars a year on them. But don't let public acceptance and fancy advertising campaigns convince you that these are effective or, even worse, harmless.

A rudimentary knowledge of physiology explains why. Our body manufactures a series of natural compounds called chondroprotective agents. These chemicals regenerate cartilage and healthy connective tissue.

Aging and overtraining, however, disrupt the body's ability to manufacture the body's own chondroprotective agents. This in turn leads to connective tissue deterioration and accompanying injury and pain.

Americans have come to rely on anti-inflammatory pain relievers, such as aspirin, acetaminophen (Advil), naploxen sodium (Aleve), and ibuprofen (Motrin). These over-the-counter drugs are all called nonsteroidal anti-inflammatory drugs (NSAIDs), and deserve their reputation as pain relievers and anti-inflammatories because they do that job.

But these quick fixes have a long-term side effect that is rarely mentioned: They inhibit cartilage repair and accelerate cartilage destruction. Connective tissue damage is caused by degeneration of cartilage; NSAIDs mask the symptoms (pain and swelling) and probably worsen the condition.

That isn't the only side effect. Athletes in particular take an added risk; taking NSAIDs before and during exercise has been linked to acute renal failure due to dehydration and stress on the kidneys. Throw in additional side effects such as gastric ulceration and liver and kidney damage, and you'll have several more reasons to wonder why "experts" and the media are so quick to label them wonder drugs.

Fortunately, there are alternatives to these remedies. European doctors, who are far more skeptical concerning the wholesale use of NSAIDs, have successfully treated osteoarthritis and other connective tissue traumas with nontoxic natural therapies for years.

One natural agent used in Europe with none of these side effects is called glucosamine. Rather than simply mask the symptoms, glucosamine treats the underlying degenerative process affecting the connective tissue. It is safe because glucosamine occurs naturally in the body as a chondroprotective agent. It stimulates the manufacture of glycosaminoglycans, which are key structural components of connective tissue.

Glucosamine also promotes the incorporation of sulfur into the connective tissue. Sulfur is a mineral that functions as an important component of connective tissue. Because of this effect, glucosamine sulfate may be the best source of glucosamine.

Supplementation may be necessary because aging or training past a certain point hinders the body's ability to manufacture sufficient levels of glucosamine. Although glucosamine is expensive and takes from four to ten weeks to produce noticeable results, clinical trials on it have been impressive. These studies compared connective tissue growth and overall physical performance in people taking glucosamine, placebos or ibuprofen.

While ibuprofen relieves pain faster, glucosamine was more successful overall. More important, it had none of ibuprofen's side effects. These results and the research behind glucosamine are so impressive that glucosamine has become the frontline therapy against osteoarthritis in Europe.

There is also reason to believe that glucosamine is an effective preventive tool. So are other natural herbal analgesics and anti-inflammatories used in Eastern medicine, such as white willow bark, ginger, tumeric, boswellia, cuercetin, bromelain, and arnica. Although the research is still ongoing, none of these products seem to have the negative consequences on connective tissue repair and growth that NSAIDs do. In addition, they each may play a beneficial role for the athlete during times of injury or trauma.

Active Recovery

Many athletes continue to train, albeit at a reduced intensity, while they have an injury. Depending on the severity of the injury, active recovery will bring much needed blood and nutrients to the injured area and help to remove metabolic waste products. Many orthopedic surgeons use both passive and active range-of-motion exercises within a day or two of certain medical procedures.

That is not to suggest that training through or immediately after an injury is necessarily a good idea. Coming back from injuries too soon often leads to compensation injuries and a constant battle to regain not only form but overall balance, since weakness or "protecting" one area leads to an injury in another. Heed the signals your body is sending you and take a day or two off. The rest may be an important aspect of training allowing your body to fully recover and gain in fitness. You will be better off following doctor's orders and taking a short time off now and avoiding the prospect of returning to the field too soon or too hard and having a major setback later.

Starting Over

Resuming an activity or a workout after you've been sidelined is always a shock because it seems like you have lost all your fitness.

Remember not to push your limits. Fitness is a process. Reevaluate your goals, be realistic, and concentrate on the small, immediate improvements you will feel. In reality, your conditioning has dropped, but it is far from where you originally started. As you will soon see, this time it will come back quicker.

16

AGING WELL IS THE BEST REVENGE

Most individuals reach their fittest levels between the ages of 20 and 30. After that, all areas of physiological fitness begin to decline. The rate each declines varies: Muscular strength and power peak in the twenties, cardiovascular endurance peaks in the early thirties. Liver and kidney functions decrease as much as 50 percent by age 70, nerve conduction velocity only declines 10 percent and cardiac output and flexibility decrease by about 20 percent. Gender differences exist as well. Men lose only about 15 percent of their bone mass by age 70 while women have lost 30 percent or more.

These age-related drops in function are difficult for every athlete—and particularly difficult for elite athletes in the public eye—to come to terms with. But there is also much to celebrate. Thanks to the more scientific approach we can now apply to training, recovery, and nutrition, athletes are extending their careers and maintaining their performance at higher levels than ever before.

Competitive Masters athletes in their 40s, 50s, and even their 60s regularly outperform recreational athletes half their age. At the 1999 **181**

United States Masters National Cycling Championships, for instance, the fastest time posted in the time trial race was by a 46-year-old competitor (beating racers 15 years younger). This is a trend that's here to stay. As a result of continued advances, the mean age of professional athletes will continue to climb in the decades to come.

It's not just elite athletes who are benefiting from these break-throughs. Although genetics will impose certain limitations, anyone can prolong and improve their performance through a more thoughtful and insightful approach to training. These scientific breakthroughs go hand in hand with our social expectations, which now encourage an aggressive approach to recreational athletics in terms of what is appropriate for a person's age.

An unhealthy diet and a sedentary lifestyle play as great, if not a greater role, than aging in the deterioration of most physiological systems and the development of most degenerative diseases. These diseases are the leading causes of death today, and although a healthy diet and exercise training won't halt the aging process, they will blunt it significantly. You don't have to have been an athlete all your life—no matter what age you begin these changes, even as late as your sixth, seventh, or eighth decade—you can still enjoy signifi-cant improvements in exercise capacity and function.

Exercise for a Long Life

We don't know for sure whether we can actually live longer because of these lifestyle changes, but several studies have shown that exercise improves longevity. In a famous Harvard alumni study of 17,000 subjects, men who expended 2,000 calories in weekly exercise had death rates one-quarter to one-third lower than classmates who did no exercise. Active individuals lived one to two years longer than their sedentary classmates. The studies' results also showed that the more exercise an individual performed per week, from 500 to 3,500 calories, the lower the risk of early death.

Although it's too early to predict the exact relationship between exercise and longevity, we already know that it enhances the quality of your life. If you train and eat properly, you can outperform sedentary 20-year-olds in terms of strength and endurance well into your 40s, 50s, or 60s. You can hold your own in endurance events against recreational athletes decades younger. More importantly, you can maintain your functional capacity (your overall or a specific physiological system's ability to perform a task) at much higher levels than others in your age group. That means that a fit 50-year-old not only has functional capacities at least 25 percent higher than a sedentary 50-year-old, but a comparable fitness level of a sedentary 20- or 30-year-old.

Nutrition and Longevity

Proper nutrition and exercise helps slow down the effects of aging. Eating a low-fat, high-fiber diet, losing weight, stopping smoking, cultivating a support system, and managing stress are all preventive measures you can take to avoid or minimize high blood pressure, high cholesterol levels, and the development of the degenerative diseases associated with aging.

As the population ages, a greater number of baby boomers and seniors are becoming increasingly interested in supplementation.

The boomers who are hitting their 50s tend to be interested in supplements that provide a youthful vitality, while seniors tend to be interested in relief from pain or chronic diseases such as heart disease and cancer.

Taking Nutrition to Heart

Certain nutritional products have been found, along with diet modification, to reduce the risk of heart disease and help to support a healthy heart. As a result of a lifelong marginal deficiency of selected micronutrients, the development of heart disease may get a stronger foothold. They include L-carnitine, co-enzyme Q10, vitamin E, and magnesium. Maintaining a healthy diet can prevent these deficiencies and at an advanced stage slow down or impede the disease's progress.

Another promising group of nutrients is the B vitamins: B_6, B_{12} and in particular, folic acid. Elevated levels of homocysteine in the blood are a risk factor for premature cardiovascular disease. Recent studies have shown that supplementation with folic acid alone, or in combination with vitamins B6 and B12, significantly reduced blood homocysteine levels and the risk of heart disease in both men and postmenopausal women.

Many cereals and other foods are now being fortified with folic acid as a result of research on folic acid deficiencies in pregnant women and birth defects. The fortification of cereals has been shown to have a positive carryover effect in decreasing heart disease risk, as well.

Cancer and Diet

While early detection methods are allowing many forms of cancer to be diagnosed earlier in life, most forms of cancer are still primarily a concern of adults in midlife and beyond. Recently the National Cancer Institute has stated that, aside from cigarette smoking, diet is the single largest cause of cancer. The National Center for Disease Control estimates that over two-thirds of all cancers are linked to preventable environmental causes, including diet.

Research studies have found several forms of cancer to be linked to diet. These include breast, colon, and prostate cancer, which are some of the leading forms of cancer and causes of cancer deaths in our society. Each of these forms of cancer has tumors that are stimulated and exasperated by the sex hormones in the body.

A low-fat, high-fiber diet is beneficial at reducing the risk of hormone dependent tumors. Reducing the fat in the diet from a typical American diet to a low-fat diet has been found to reduce cancer risk by as much as 30 percent. Adding fiber to the diet helps to increase estrogen excretion in the feces and lower both blood estrogen levels and hormone dependent cancer risk. For this reason the American Cancer Society, along with other organizations, recommends a daily fiber intake of 20 to 35 grams per day.

The use of soy products has also been linked to a reduced cancer risk. In particular the isoflavone genistein has proven beneficial in reducing cancer risk. Not only is genistein found in tofu and soy beans, but is present in most isolated soy protein products. These powders can be used in cooking and in shakes to help supplement the diet with a low-fat protein source that carries positive health benefits.

Several herbs have been used in the treatment of benign prosta-tic hypertrophy (BPH), a noncancerous enlargement of the prostate. This enlargement is often painful and can be a precursor to prostate cancer.

Saw palmetto berry extract, pygeum, and pumpkin seed have all been effective in reducing the symptoms and clinical signs of BPH, primarily because they block sex-hormone receptors and the conver-sion of testosterone in the prostate. These herbs appear to be as, if not more, effective as prescription medications, but without the neg-ative side effects.

Aging and Weight Gain

You don't need a book to tell you that most people gain weight as they get older. It is not uncommon for individuals in our society to gain weight as they age. Not only is there an age-related increase in body weight; there is also an increase in body fat and decrease in lean muscle.

Physical activity certainly helps to thwart these changes. The more time someone spends exercising, the lower their body-fat lev-els tend to be, so a sedentary lifestyle is part of the culprit for this increase in weight. In addition, the typical American diet—high in fat and calories and reliant on processed foods—also plays a role.

But aging, too, might be to blame. There appears to be some increase in body weight that is independent of activity level as we age. In a study on 7,000 male runners, regular endurance exercise at a constant intensity level did not totally blunt the tendency for adults to add weight as they get older.

In other studies, people who exercised less had greater gains in weight than those who exercised more. As body weight and body fat go up when people age, muscle mass goes down. Because the amount of lean muscle mass is one of the primary factors that affects your metabolism and the number of calories you can take in to maintain your body weight, as muscle mass goes down, so too must calories.

Perhaps the best way to retain muscle mass as you age is to incorporate strength, or resistance, training into your workout schedule. While cardiovascular endurance exercise burns calories and fat, it won't systematically maintain enough muscle mass. Weight training is the only solution.

The maintenance of muscle mass is critical for body weight regulation. For this reason the ACSM, and others, recommend weight training along with aerobic exercise for maintenance of a preferable body composition, weight management, and the drop in function, performance, and muscle mass associated with aging.

Rehydration and Aging

Rehydration after exercise is of particular concern with regards to aging since the thirst drive weakens with age. Because of this lower thirst drive, elderly people do not recover from dehydration as quickly as younger athletes. This chronic state of dehydration may diminish cardiac function, limit optimal performance, and even explain less than optimal blood volume in the elderly.

Requirements for rehydration do not change as we get older, maintaining hydration—even if it takes an extra effort to do so—is imperative, because it can improve exercise performance and recovery.

The Fountain of Youth

Proper diet and exercise do counteract many of the effects of premature aging brought on by the typical American diet and lifestyle. That doesn't mean you are going to look like a teenager or live to be past 100. But you will function like someone decades younger, beat kids half your age, and play with your grandchildren all day long. Along the way, you'll be a real inspiration to the people who matter to you.

PART V

PERSONAL BEST—
A PROGRAM JUST FOR YOU

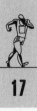

17

YOU ARE WHAT YOU EAT

The *Fuel Up* program has been designed to allow you to personalize your daily nutritional and dietary requirements based on your body weight and training level. The program includes a diet diary, which you will use to calculate your daily nutrient and caloric intakes.

Using the tables provided and factoring in your daily workout, you will determine your nutrient and caloric recommendations for that day. Your daily nutrient intake and total calories will vary dramatically from day to day, depending on your daily workouts.

Because the two most important nutrients for performance and recovery are carbohydrates and proteins, each of these nutrients will be calculated individually. Based on your carbohydrate and protein recommendations, you will then determine your fat intake for that day. It will be set at a level of 10 or 20 percent of your total caloric intake depending upon your goals. Because saturated fat has so many negative effects on health and performance, I recommend you limit your saturated-fat intake to less than 5 percent of your total calories.

To determine the amount of each macronutrient in the foods you eat, use either the information from the labels on the foods themselves, from the values in Appendix III (p. 233), or the average ballpark values table provided later in this chapter. To help you maintain optimal hydration throughout the day as well as during and after training, a hydration diary (p. 229) is also provided.

Using these diaries is the most effective way to keep an accurate record of what you eat. This might seem tedious and time consuming at first, but with practice it will become second nature. Because many of the meals you eat will be similar in content, you won't have to do the calculations every time. By maintaining it, you will be able to look back over your previous diaries to discover any weak links in your nutritional program that may be limiting your overall progress.

The Diary Works

By keeping track not only of your training, but also of your diet, you can quickly spot strengths and weaknesses in your program. Wes and Gina are two clients who found the diary helpful in charting their progress, particularly in the early phases of their training.

Wes, who is in his early 50s, had missed the previous year's competitive cycling season for work-related reasons. In the year off, he had gained quite a bit of unwanted weight. Being impatient with a slow but steady loss in body fat and weight, he decided against his better judgment to go on one of the popular, high-protein, low-carbohydrate diets.

Initially, he was ecstatic with the results of his weight loss, training, and performance. He hadn't ridden regularly in more than a year and felt his fitness progressively improve now that he was riding five to six days a week. With his rapid weight loss, he could climb the hills with greater ease.

However, after a month he noticed that although he had dropped almost 15 pounds, his performance was no longer improving. Moreover, he had no energy toward the end of his rides and often struggled to make it home. Although he had lost a significant amount of weight and was within two or three pounds of his desired "racing weight," he was no longer able to match the power or speed of the other riders. Not only had his energy levels dropped, his motivation was also flagging.

After we looked at his diary, the problems quickly became apparent. First, Wes was only taking in 50 to 70 grams of carbohydrates per day. This was the amount he should be taking in on each ride, not each day. Once we changed his carbohydrate intake to 350 to 500 grams per day, depending on his workout intensity, his progress was renewed, and he was able to drop another two pounds.

The diary also revealed that he had been drinking but not eating during the workout. I suggested that he eat an energy bar with 40 grams of carbohydrates for every hour on the bike. This, combined with his fluid intake, let him last longer and push harder on the training rides and in races. He quickly regained his form and confidence, continued to train with the Masters World Championships as his goal, and ended up with a top-20 finish in his category.

Twenty-seven-year-old Gina's problems were just the opposite of Wes's. Although she was taking in an appropriate level of calories for a slow weight and fat loss, she was eating a low-fat diet based primarily on carbohydrates. Although she took three fitness classes a week and ran or walked with a friend two other days, she didn't think of herself as an athlete and felt she didn't need to eat like one.

She may not have been a competitive athlete, but she was still placing stress on her system. Despite her apparently healthful lifestyle, she was chronically tired and increasingly prone to various respiratory infections and minor, nagging aches and pains.

I convinced her to keep a diary, so she could see for herself that she was eating enough protein for a sedentary person, but only one quarter to one half of what she needed based on her activity levels. The process of keeping the diary helped convince her that she needed to eat more protein. Once she did, Gina found that her overall sense of wellness improved and that her exercise regimen was more enjoyable. The extra protein enhanced her immune system and resulted in pain-free workouts.

Personalizing Your Program

Personalizing caloric recommendations to fit your own needs is very simple. The nutrient recommendations are determined by the difficulty of your workouts and in particular by the combination of the workout intensity and duration. First, you'll figure out how much and how hard you work out. After evaluating the difficulty of your workout, you'll calculate the exact recommended intakes of carbohydrates and protein necessary for optimal adaptations based upon that training load and your body weight.

After these two nutrient levels are determined, you'll select your fat intake based on 10 to 20 percent of your total calories. If you are interested in weight loss or maintenance or are exercising for relatively short periods of time, you can have adequate energy (calories) with 10 percent fat, combined with appropriate protein and carbohydrate intakes. If you're involved in endurance exercise and particularly if you are working out longer than two hours a day, up the percentage toward the 20 percent limit. The tables and diaries in this section will assist you in determining your precise intake levels.

Nutrient-Intake Levels

Tables One through Three provide the recommended daily carbohydrate, protein, and fat intakes based upon your body weight and training intensity level. Using these values, you will be able to select foods that meet these requirements.

Table One on page 200 lists the recommended daily carbohydrate intake based upon exercise intensity levels for body weights ranging from 100 to 250 pounds. The values are given in two-pound increments. If your body weight is not listed, use the equation at the end of the table to calculate the exact amount of carbohydrates you need each day. To find out your protein requirements, repeat the process using Table Two on page 204, which lists recommended daily protein intake.

Once you have determined your carbohydrate and protein recommendations, you can use Table Three on page 207 to discover your desired daily total fat intake. The table has been arranged to not only list recommendations based upon exercise intensity, but has also been subcategorized to include intake levels of either 10 or 20 percent of fat relative to total calories.

The level of fat recommended in *Fuel Up*, set at either 10 or 20 percent of the total caloric intake, meets or exceeds the recommended guidelines for health established by the most important organizations, such as the American College of Sports Medicine, the American Council on Exercise, the American Medical Association, the American Cancer Society, and the American Diabetes Association. In addition, the nutritional regimen that results in optimal performance is also the best diet for health and disease prevention.

The Hydration Diary on page 229 will enable you to follow both the generalized hydration guidelines along with your specific needs dependent upon your training regimen. Complete each section, placing a check to signify the amount you drink. Once you have completed your exercise hydration and rehydration, determine your overall nutrient intakes from the fluids ingested and list them on the section at the bottom of the page.

Finally, insert the information from Tables One through Three into the desired nutrient intake row of your Daily Diet Diary on page 231. These levels will be your goals and will determine your food intake for the day. Throughout each day, complete the diary using the sections for your meals and snacks along with the specific section to record your exercise intake. Using the diary helps you plan your shopping and menus days in advance.

Intensity and Body Weight Matter

So how do you define your workout's intensity? Low-intensity exercise is characterized by exercise performed relatively easily (50 to 60 percent of maximal heart rate for cardiovascular activities or 60 to 70 percent of maximal strength capacity during resistance training or other anaerobic activities) for less than an hour. These types of activities include lifting light weights, playing an easy game of tennis, or jogging at a leisurely pace, possibly a recovery workout interspersed between hard-workout days. Exercise performed for more than one hour below your target heart rate also falls into the low-intensity category.

Moderate-intensity workouts are those in which you work at a moderate to high intensity (70 to 85 percent of your maximal heart rate in aerobic activities or 70 to 80 percent of your maximal strength capacity for anaerobic activities) for less than an hour or at the low end of these intensity ranges for workouts greater than an hour. High-intensity workouts include those undertaken by people initiating new training programs at any intensity level, those increasing their overall training load, those whose workouts are longer than two hours, or those who are performing at maximum work loads for sessions less than two hours.

Once you determine which category your training for the day falls under, you will be able to identify your nutrient intake level for each macronutrient. Remember that the level will change from day to day, according to the duration and intensity of your training. Your overall caloric intake will also change, necessitating a program that must be adjusted daily.

A New Kind of Calorie Counting

Sam, 29, and Aida, 27, are both active and athletic. One weekend they went to the country club. Sam played nine holes of golf on the executive course, while Aida played five intense sets of tennis in a club tournament. Sam weighs 50 pounds more than Aida, but on this day he needed less total calories and one-quarter less protein for his activities than she did to have enough fuel for her activities.

The explanation can be found in the difference between their training intensities for the day. Although Sam walked the nine holes and was out on the course for two hours, his training intensity was relatively low and the total distance he covered was just under two miles. Aida, on the other hand, played high-intensity, competitive tennis for close to three hours. She burned so many more nutrients and calories that she had to out eat Sam if she was to recover.

	AIDA		SAM	
Bodyweight	128 pounds		186 pounds	
Carbohydrates	582 grams (10.0 g/kg BW)	2,328 Calories (4 kcal/gram)	592 grams (7.0 g/kg BW)	2,368 Calories (4 kcal/gram)
Protein	116 grams (2.0 g/kg BW)	464 Calories (4 kcal/gram)	85 grams (1.0 g/kg BW)	340 Calories (4 kcal/gram)
Fat (@ 10% Kcals)	34 grams	306 Calories	33 grams	297 Calories
Total Calories		3,098 Calories		3,005 Calories

Things changed the next day. Sam went to the gym for a heavy, weight workout and a half-hour run on the treadmill. This was a hard-training day and required a much higher nutrient intake level.

He needed to eat 845 grams of carbohydrate, 169 grams of protein, and 50 grams of fat. His total caloric intake of 4,506 calories was also 50 percent higher than the previous day's.

Aida, who took the day off, found herself at the opposite end of the training spectrum. Because she expended less calories she saw her nutrient intake dip to 407 grams of carbohydrate, 58 grams of protein, and 23 grams of fat for a total caloric intake of 2,062 calories. This was 35 percent fewer calories than the day before.

It's interesting to note that because nutrient intakes vary depending on your workout intensity, a lighter individual will often require higher levels of specific nutrients than someone nearly twice their size.

Tables of Recommended Daily Nutrient Intakes

Tables One through Three denote the desired daily carbohydrate, protein, and fat intakes based upon your body weight and exercise training intensity. Use these tables to determine both your daily nutrient intake levels in grams and your total daily calorie intake level. Each row contains the grams and calories for your selected body weight based upon your workout intensity for that day. Write down the gram and calorie values for each nutrient and then transfer the individual gram values and the total of all three caloric values onto your diet diary. These values are your day's nutrient intake guidelines.

For the sake of convenience, Table Four on page 211 presents a summary of the daily nutrient intake levels for protein, carbohydrate, and fat, along with the daily caloric intake level, for selected body weights from 100 to 250 pounds in 25-pound increments. You can use this table if your body weight meets one of the set levels or to check your values from Tables One to Three.

See Appendix III, "Nutritive Values for Selected Foods" (page 233), to match your carbohydrate, protein, and fat requirements with your daily diet.

TABLE ONE

Recommendations for Daily Carbohydrate Intake

BODY WEIGHT (LBS.)	LOW INTENSITY (G/DAY)	(KCAL)	MODERATE INTENSITY (G/DAY)	(KCAL)	HIGH INTENSITY (G/DAY)	(KCAL)
100	318	1,273	386	1,544	455	1,820
102	325	1,300	394	1,576	464	1,856
104	331	1,324	402	1,608	473	1,892
106	337	1,348	410	1,640	482	1,928
108	344	1,376	417	1,668	491	1,964
110	350	1,400	425	1,700	500	2,000
112	356	1,424	433	1,732	509	2,036
114	363	1,452	440	1,760	518	2,072
116	369	1,476	448	1,792	527	2,108
118	375	1,500	456	1,824	536	2,144
120	382	1,528	464	1,856	545	2,180
122	388	1,552	471	1,884	555	2,220
124	395	1,580	479	1,916	564	2,256
126	401	1,604	487	1,948	573	2,292
128	407	1,628	495	1,980	582	2,328
130	414	1,656	502	2,008	591	2,364

BODY WEIGHT (LBS.)	LOW INTENSITY		MODERATE INTENSITY		HIGH INTENSITY	
	(G/DAY)	(KCAL)	(G/DAY)	(KCAL)	(G/DAY)	(KCAL)
132	420	1,680	510	2,040	600	2,400
134	426	1,704	518	2,072	609	2,436
136	433	1,732	525	2,100	618	2,472
138	439	1,756	533	2,132	627	2,508
140	445	1,780	541	2,164	636	2,544
142	452	1,808	549	2,196	645	2,580
144	458	1,832	556	2,224	655	2,620
146	465	1,860	564	2,256	664	2,656
148	471	1,884	572	2,288	673	2,692
150	477	1,908	580	2,320	682	2,728
152	484	1,936	587	2,348	691	2,764
154	490	1,960	595	2,380	700	2,800
156	496	1,984	603	2,412	709	2,836
158	503	2,012	610	2,440	718	2,872
160	509	2,036	618	2,472	727	2,908
162	515	2,060	626	2,504	736	2,944
164	522	2,088	634	2,536	745	2,980
166	528	2,112	641	2,564	755	3,020
168	535	2,140	649	2,596	764	3,054
170	541	2,164	657	2,628	773	3,092
172	547	2,188	665	2,660	782	3,128
174	554	2,216	672	2,688	791	3,164
176	560	2,240	680	2,720	800	3,200
178	566	2,264	688	2,752	809	3,236
180	573	2,292	695	2,780	818	3,272
182	579	2,316	703	2,812	827	3,308

continued

BODY WEIGHT (LBS.)	LOW INTENSITY		MODERATE INTENSITY		HIGH INTENSITY	
	(G/DAY)	(KCAL)	(G/DAY)	(KCAL)	(G/DAY)	(KCAL)
184	585	2,340	711	2,844	836	3,344
186	592	2,368	719	2,876	845	3,380
188	598	2,392	726	2,904	855	3,420
190	**605**	**2,420**	**734**	**2,936**	**864**	**3,456**
192	611	2,444	742	2,968	873	3,492
194	617	2,468	750	3,000	882	3,528
196	624	2,496	757	3,028	891	3,564
198	630	2,520	765	3,060	900	3,600
200	**636**	**2,544**	**773**	**3,092**	**909**	**3,636**
202	643	2,572	780	3,120	918	3,672
204	649	2,596	788	3,152	927	3,708
206	655	2,620	796	3,184	936	3,744
208	662	2,648	804	3,216	945	3,780
210	**668**	**2,672**	**811**	**3,244**	**955**	**3,820**
212	675	2,700	819	3,276	964	3,856
214	681	2,724	827	3,308	973	3,892
216	687	2,748	835	3,340	982	3,928
218	694	2,776	842	3,368	991	3,964
220	**700**	**2,800**	**850**	**3,400**	**1,000**	**4,000**
222	706	2,824	858	3,432	1,009	4,036
224	713	2,852	865	3,460	1,018	4,072
226	719	2,876	873	3,492	1,027	4,108
228	725	2,900	881	3,524	1,036	4,144
230	**732**	**2,928**	**889**	**3,556**	**1,045**	**4,180**
232	738	2,952	896	3,584	1,055	4,220
234	745	2,980	904	3,616	1,064	4,256

BODY WEIGHT (LBS.)	LOW INTENSITY		MODERATE INTENSITY		HIGH INTENSITY	
	(G/DAY)	(KCAL)	(G/DAY)	(KCAL)	(G/DAY)	(KCAL)
236	751	3,004	912	3,648	1,073	4,292
238	757	3,028	920	3,680	1,082	4,328
240	**764**	**3,056**	**927**	**3,708**	**1,091**	**4,364**
242	770	3,080	935	3,740	1,100	4,400
244	776	3,104	943	3,772	1,109	4,436
246	783	3,132	950	3,800	1,118	4,472
248	789	3,156	958	3,832	1,127	4,508
250	**795**	**3,180**	**966**	**3,864**	**1,136**	**4,544**

If your body weight is not listed in Table One, you can use one of the following equations to determine your individual daily carbohydrate requirement. Values have been rounded to the nearest whole number. Daily carbohydrate recommendations based on training intensity levels and body weight are as follows: Low Intensity – 7.0 g/kg/day, Moderate Intensity – 8.5 g/kg/day, and High Intensity – 10.0g/kg/day.

Low Intensity:

_____ / (2.2 kg/lb) × (7.0 g/kg/day) = _____ g/day × 4 Cal/g = _____ Calories.
Body weight

Moderate Intensity:

_____ / (2.2 kg/lb) × (8.5 g/kg/day) = _____ g/day × 4 Cal/g = _____ Calories.
Body weight

High Intensity:

_____ / (2.2 kg/lb) × (10.0 g/kg/day) = _____ g/day × 4 Cal/g = _____ Calories.
Body weight

TABLE TWO

Recommendations for Daily Protein Intake

BODY WEIGHT (LBS.)	LOW INTENSITY (G/DAY)	(KCAL)	MODERATE INTENSITY (G/DAY)	(KCAL)	HIGH INTENSITY (G/DAY)	(KCAL)
100	45	180	68	272	91	364
102	46	184	70	280	93	372
104	47	188	71	284	95	380
106	48	192	72	288	96	384
108	49	196	74	296	98	392
110	50	200	75	300	100	400
112	51	204	76	304	102	408
114	52	208	78	312	104	416
116	53	212	79	316	105	420
118	54	216	80	320	107	428
120	55	220	82	328	109	436
122	55	220	83	332	111	444
124	56	224	85	340	113	452
126	57	228	86	344	115	460
128	58	232	87	348	116	464
130	59	236	89	356	118	472
132	60	240	90	360	120	480
134	61	244	91	364	122	488
136	62	248	93	372	124	496
138	63	252	94	376	125	500
140	64	256	95	380	127	508
142	65	260	97	388	129	516

BODY WEIGHT (LBS.)	LOW INTENSITY (G/DAY)	(KCAL)	MODERATE INTENSITY (G/DAY)	(KCAL)	HIGH INTENSITY (G/DAY)	(KCAL)
144	65	260	98	392	131	524
146	66	264	100	400	133	532
148	67	268	101	404	135	540
150	68	272	102	408	136	544
152	69	276	104	416	138	552
154	70	280	105	420	140	560
156	71	284	106	424	142	568
158	72	288	108	432	144	576
160	73	292	109	436	145	580
162	74	296	110	440	147	588
164	75	300	112	448	149	596
166	75	300	113	452	151	604
168	76	304	115	460	153	612
170	77	308	116	464	155	620
172	78	312	117	468	156	624
174	79	316	119	476	158	632
176	80	320	120	480	160	640
178	81	324	121	484	162	648
180	82	328	123	492	164	656
182	83	332	124	496	165	660
184	84	336	125	500	167	668
186	85	340	127	508	169	676
188	85	340	128	512	171	684
190	86	344	130	520	173	692
192	87	348	131	524	175	700
194	88	352	132	528	176	704

continued

BODY WEIGHT (LBS.)	LOW INTENSITY		MODERATE INTENSITY		HIGH INTENSITY	
	(G/DAY)	(KCAL)	(G/DAY)	(KCAL)	(G/DAY)	(KCAL)
196	89	356	134	536	178	712
198	90	360	135	540	180	720
200	91	364	136	544	182	728
202	92	366	138	552	184	736
204	93	372	139	556	185	740
206	94	376	140	560	187	748
208	95	380	142	568	189	756
210	95	380	143	572	191	764
212	96	384	145	580	193	772
214	97	388	146	584	195	780
216	98	392	147	588	196	784
218	99	396	149	596	198	792
220	100	400	150	600	200	800
222	101	404	151	604	202	808
224	102	408	153	612	204	816
226	103	412	154	616	205	820
228	104	416	155	620	207	828
230	105	420	157	628	209	836
232	105	420	158	632	211	844
234	106	424	160	640	213	852
236	107	428	161	644	215	860
238	108	432	162	648	216	864
240	109	436	164	656	218	872
242	110	440	165	660	220	880
244	111	444	166	664	222	888

BODY WEIGHT (LBS.)	LOW INTENSITY (G/DAY)	(KCAL)	MODERATE INTENSITY (G/DAY)	(KCAL)	HIGH INTENSITY (G/DAY)	(KCAL)
246	112	448	168	672	224	896
248	113	452	169	676	225	900
250	114	456	170	680	227	908

If your body weight is not listed in Table Two, you can use one of the following equations to determine your individual daily protein requirement. Values have been rounded to the nearest whole number. Daily protein recommendations based on training intensity levels and body weight are as follows: Low Intensity – 1.0 g/kg/day, Moderate Intensity – 1.5 g/kg/day, and High Intensity – 2.0g/kg/day.

Low Intensity:

_____ / (2.2 kg/lb) × (1.0 g/kg/day) = _____ g/day × 4 Cal/g = _____ Calories.
Body weight

Moderate Intensity:

_____ / (2.2 kg/lb) × (1.5 g/kg/day) = _____ g/day × 4 Cal/g = _____ Calories.
Body weight

High Intensity:

_____ / (2.2 kg/lb) × (2.0 g/kg/day) = _____ g/day × 4 Cal/g = _____ Calories.
Body weight

TABLE THREE

Recommendations for Daily Fat Intake

BODY WEIGHT (lbs.)	LOW INTENSITY @ 10% (g/day) (kcal)		@ 20% (g/day) (kcal)		MODERATE INTENSITY @ 10% (g/day) (kcal)		@20% (g/day) (kcal)		HIGH INTENSITY @ 10% (g/day) (kcal)		@20% (g/day) (kcal)	
100	18	162	41	369	22	198	51	459	27	243	61	549
102	18	162	42	378	23	207	52	468	27	243	62	558

continued

BODY WEIGHT	LOW INTENSITY				MODERATE INTENSITY				HIGH INTENSITY			
	@ 10%		@ 20%		@ 10%		@20%		@ 10%		@20%	
(lbs.)	(g/day)	(kcal)	(g/day)	(kcal)	(g/day)	(kcal)	(g/day)	(kcal)	(g/day)	(kcal)	(g/day)	(kcal)
104	19	171	42	378	23	207	53	477	28	252	64	576
106	19	171	43	387	24	216	54	486	28	252	65	585
108	19	171	44	396	24	216	55	495	29	261	66	594
110	**20**	**180**	**45**	**405**	**25**	**225**	**56**	**504**	**29**	**261**	**67**	**603**
112	20	180	46	414	25	225	57	513	30	270	68	612
114	20	180	46	414	25	225	58	522	30	270	70	630
116	21	189	47	423	26	234	59	531	31	279	71	639
118	21	189	48	432	26	234	60	540	32	288	72	648
120	**21**	**189**	**49**	**441**	**27**	**243**	**61**	**549**	**32**	**288**	**73**	**657**
122	22	198	50	450	27	243	62	558	33	297	75	675
124	22	198	51	459	28	252	63	567	33	297	76	684
126	22	198	51	459	28	252	64	576	34	306	77	693
128	23	207	52	468	29	261	65	585	34	306	78	702
130	**23**	**207**	**53**	**477**	**29**	**261**	**66**	**594**	**35**	**315**	**79**	**711**
132	24	216	54	486	29	261	67	603	35	315	81	729
134	24	216	55	495	30	270	68	612	36	324	82	738
136	24	216	55	495	30	270	69	621	36	324	83	747
138	25	225	56	504	31	279	70	630	37	333	84	756
140	**25**	**225**	**57**	**513**	**31**	**279**	**71**	**639**	**37**	**333**	**86**	**774**
142	25	225	58	522	32	288	72	648	38	342	87	783
144	26	234	59	531	32	288	73	657	38	342	88	792
146	26	234	59	531	33	297	74	666	39	351	89	801
148	26	234	60	540	33	297	75	675	40	360	90	810
150	**27**	**243**	**61**	**549**	**33**	**297**	**76**	**684**	**40**	**360**	**92**	**828**
152	27	243	62	558	34	306	77	693	41	369	93	837
154	27	243	63	567	34	306	78	702	41	369	94	846

BODY WEIGHT (lbs.)	LOW INTENSITY				MODERATE INTENSITY				HIGH INTENSITY			
	@ 10%		@ 20%		@ 10%		@20%		@ 10%		@20%	
	(g/day)	(kcal)	(g/day)	(kcal)	(g/day)	(kcal)	(g/day)	(kcal)	(g/day)	(kcal)	(g/day)	(kcal)
156	28	252	64	576	35	315	79	711	42	378	95	855
158	28	252	64	576	35	315	80	720	42	378	97	873
160	**29**	**261**	**65**	**585**	**36**	**324**	**81**	**729**	**43**	**387**	**98**	**882**
162	29	261	66	594	36	324	82	738	43	387	99	891
164	29	261	67	603	37	333	83	747	44	396	100	900
166	30	270	68	612	37	333	85	765	44	396	101	909
168	30	270	68	612	37	333	86	774	45	405	103	927
170	**30**	**270**	**69**	**621**	**38**	**342**	**87**	**783**	**45**	**405**	**104**	**936**
172	31	279	70	630	38	342	88	792	46	414	105	945
174	31	279	71	639	39	351	89	801	47	423	106	954
176	31	279	72	648	39	351	90	810	47	423	108	972
178	32	288	72	648	40	360	91	819	48	432	109	981
180	**32**	**288**	**73**	**657**	**40**	**360**	**92**	**828**	**48**	**432**	**110**	**990**
182	32	288	74	666	41	369	93	837	49	441	111	999
184	33	297	75	675	41	369	94	846	49	441	112	1,008
186	33	297	76	684	41	369	95	855	50	450	114	1,026
188	33	297	77	693	42	378	96	864	50	450	115	1,035
190	**34**	**306**	**77**	**693**	**42**	**378**	**97**	**873**	**51**	**459**	**116**	**1,044**
192	34	306	78	702	43	387	98	882	51	459	117	1,053
194	35	315	79	711	43	387	99	891	52	468	119	1,071
196	35	315	80	720	44	396	100	900	52	468	120	1,080
198	35	315	81	729	44	396	101	909	53	477	121	1,019
200	**36**	**324**	**81**	**729**	**45**	**405**	**102**	**918**	**53**	**477**	**122**	**1,098**
202	36	324	82	738	45	405	103	927	54	486	123	1,107
204	36	324	83	747	45	405	104	936	55	495	125	1,125
206	37	333	84	756	46	414	105	945	55	495	126	1,134

continued

BODY WEIGHT (lbs.)	LOW INTENSITY @ 10% (g/day)	(kcal)	@ 20% (g/day)	(kcal)	MODERATE INTENSITY @ 10% (g/day)	(kcal)	@20% (g/day)	(kcal)	HIGH INTENSITY @ 10% (g/day)	(kcal)	@20% (g/day)	(kcal)
208	37	333	85	765	46	414	106	954	56	504	127	1,143
210	37	333	86	774	47	423	107	963	56	504	128	1,152
212	38	342	86	774	47	423	108	972	57	513	130	1,170
214	38	342	87	783	48	432	109	981	57	513	131	1,179
216	38	342	88	792	48	432	110	990	58	522	132	1,188
218	39	351	89	801	49	441	111	999	58	522	133	1,197
220	39	351	90	810	49	441	112	1,008	59	531	134	1,206
222	40	360	90	810	49	441	113	1,017	59	531	136	1,224
224	40	360	91	819	50	450	114	1,026	60	540	137	1,233
226	40	360	92	828	50	450	115	1,035	60	540	138	1,242
228	41	369	93	837	51	459	116	1,044	61	549	139	1,251
230	41	369	94	846	51	459	117	1,053	61	549	141	1,269
232	41	369	94	846	52	468	118	1,062	62	558	142	1,278
234	42	378	95	855	52	468	119	1,071	63	567	143	1,287
236	42	378	96	864	53	477	120	1,080	63	567	144	1,296
238	42	378	97	873	53	477	121	1,089	64	576	145	1,305
240	43	387	98	882	53	477	122	1,098	64	576	147	1,323
242	43	387	99	891	54	486	123	1,107	65	585	148	1,332
244	43	387	99	891	54	486	124	1,116	65	585	149	1,341
246	44	396	100	900	55	495	125	1,125	66	594	150	1,350
248	44	396	101	909	55	495	126	1,134	66	594	152	1,368
250	45	405	102	918	56	504	127	1,143	67	603	153	1,377

If your body weight is not listed in Table Three, you can use one of the following equations to determine your individual daily fat recommendation. Values have been rounded to the nearest whole number. Daily fat recommendations are based on either an overall dietary fat intake of 10 or 20 percent of your total daily caloric intake.

@ 10 percent of total calories from fat:

(_____ + _____) × (0.049) = _____ g/day × 9 Cal/g = _____ Calories.
Grams   Grams
Protein   Carbohydrate

@ 20 percent of total calories from fat:

(_____ + _____) × (0.112) = _____ g/day × 9 Cal/g = _____ Calories.
Grams   Grams
Protein   Carbohydrate

TABLE FOUR

Overall Daily Nutrient Intake Recommendations

	LOW INTENSITY (GRAMS / DAY)	MODERATE INTENSITY (GRAMS / DAY)	HIGH INTENSITY (GRAMS / DAY)
100 lb. Athlete			
Carbohydrate	318	386	455
Protein	45	68	91
Fat @ 10% of calories	18	22	27
@ 20% of calories	41	51	61
Total Daily Calories			
@ 10% Dietary Fat	1,614	2,014	2,427
@ 20% Dietary Fat	1,821	2,275	2,733
125 lb. Athlete			
Carbohydrate	398	483	568
Protein	57	85	114
Fat @ 10% of calories	22	28	33
@ 20% of calories	51	64	76
Total Daily Calories			
@ 10% Dietary Fat	2,018	2,524	3,025
@ 20% Dietary Fat	2,279	2,848	3,412

continued

	LOW INTENSITY (GRAMS / DAY)	MODERATE INTENSITY (GRAMS / DAY)	HIGH INTENSITY (GRAMS / DAY)
150 lb. Athlete			
Carbohydrate	477	580	682
Protein	68	102	136
Fat @ 10% of calories	27	33	40
@ 20% of calories	61	76	92
Total Daily Calories			
@ 10% Dietary Fat	2,423	3,025	3,632
@ 20% Dietary Fat	2,729	3,412	4,100
175 lb. Athlete			
Carbohydrate	557	676	795
Protein	80	119	159
Fat @ 10% of calories	31	39	47
@ 20% of calories	71	89	107
Total Daily Calories			
@ 10% Dietary Fat	2,827	3,531	4,239
@ 20% Dietary Fat	3,187	3,981	4,779
200 lb. Athlete			
Carbohydrate	636	773	909
Protein	91	136	182
Fat @ 10% of calories	36	45	53
@ 20% of calories	81	102	122
Total Daily Calories			
@ 10% Dietary Fat	3,232	4,041	4,841
@ 20% Dietary Fat	3,637	4,554	5,462
250 lb. Athlete			
Carbohydrate	795	966	1,136
Protein	114	170	227
Fat @ 10% of calories	45	56	67
@ 20% of calories	102	127	153
Total Daily Calories			
@ 10% Dietary Fat	4,041	5,048	6,055
@ 20% Dietary Fat	4,554	5,687	6,829

Ballpark Figures of Nutrient Values

Often when you are eating out, you don't have a book with the nutrient values of food with you nor are they listed on the menu. Below is a table that presents average nutrient values for selected food groups. Although using these values is not as precise as determining the actual value of each food, they provide a ballpark estimate of a meal's or day's nutrient content. You can make a copy of this table to use when you are eating out to gauge the nutrient intake of your meal.

AVERAGE NUTRIENT CONTENT OF FOOD GROUPS

	PROTEIN (GRAMS)	CARBOHYDRATE (GRAMS)	FAT (GRAMS)	CALORIES
Meats:				
low-fat (lean)	7	0	3	55
medium-fat	7	0	5	75
high-fat	7	0	8	100
Dairy:				
skim, nonfat	8	12	0	90
low-fat	8	12	5	120
whole fat	8	12	8	150
Grains/Vegetables	2–3	2–15	0–2	50–90
Fruit	0	15	0	60

Now that you've seen the averages for each category, let's break it down. An easy way to figure out how much protein you are having in a meal is to remember that there are an average of seven grams of protein per ounce of animal protein (meat), eight grams of protein per serving of dairy, and two to three grams of protein per serving of carbohydrate.

The caloric content of meat and dairy protein sources will vary depending on the fat content. In general, a four-ounce serving is about the size of an average palm. Most "sit down" restaurants define a portion's size of meat as between eight and twelve ounces.

Meat products can be separated based on their fat content. Low-fat or lean meats, which contain approximately 7 grams of protein, also provide three or less grams of fat and approximately 55 calories per ounce. Included in this category of low-fat meats are USDA choice cuts of lean beef, lean pork, and veal, poultry without the skin, most types of fish, and luncheon meats that are 95 to 99 percent fat free. Egg whites also fall into the low-fat category because they contain no fat or carbohydrate, three grams of protein and 15 calories per egg white.

Medium-fat meats contain 5 grams of fat and 75 calories per ounce and include most cuts of beef such as ground beef, porterhouse steak, and rump roast; pork chops and cutlets, veal chops and roast, poultry with skin, salmon, sole, mackerel, luncheon meats that are 86 to 94 percent fat-free, and one whole egg.

High-fat meats contain 8 grams of fat and 100 calories per ounce and include USDA Prime cuts of beef and pork including ribs, ground pork, ground lamb, fried fish and most luncheon meats, sausages, and hot dogs. Most whole-fat cheeses from the dairy category are also considered high fat.

For dairy products one serving, which equals one cup, or eight ounces, contains 12 grams of carbohydrate and eight grams of protein. The calorie and fat content will vary from negligible amounts of fat and 90 calories per serving for skim/nonfat dairy products to 5 grams of fat and 120 calories for low-fat dairy products to up to 8 grams and 150 calories for whole-fat dairy products.

A serving of fruit, grains, or vegetable will vary from ⅓ to ½ a cup for most beans and grains to ½ cup for cooked vegetables and one cup for many fresh vegetables. Fruits and processed sugars contain negligible amounts of protein, and most grains, vegetables, and fruits also contain negligible amounts of fat. The carbohydrate content of these foods range from 2 to 15 grams per cup. Some exceptions include avocados, olives, and coconuts, all of which contain minute amounts of carbohydrates and protein and about five grams of fat per serving. Another exception is soybeans, which contain 120 calories, 10 grams of protein, 8 grams of carbohydrate and 5 grams of fat per serving.

Menus for Success

Thirty-two-year-old Kimberly has decided to enter a half-marathon with a friend. She has three months to train and wants to finish the half-marathon in around two hours. Although she is already in excellent shape, she has had to add mileage and step up the intensity of her training. She has also had to change her diet.

Because she has a family, she has to work out first thing every day. Sundays are her long-run day, with an eventual goal of running for two hours. Mondays are devoted to a short recovery run. Tuesdays she walks with her daughter in the morning and takes a yoga class in the late afternoon or early evening. Wednesday and Thursdays she runs four to five miles, with an additional yoga class on Thursdays. On Fridays she walks or jogs. On Saturdays she runs another four to five miles.

Because Kimberly is changing intensities and distances almost every day, her nutritional requirements will vary from day to day. She weighs 125 pounds, which is appropriate for her size and fitness level. Because she is not trying to lose weight, her fat intake level is set at 20 percent on hard-workout days and 10 percent on the others.

Kimberly needs to take in 568 grams of carbohydrates, 114 grams of protein, and 75 grams of fat totaling 3,403 calories on hard-workout days. On these days her diet is approximately 67 percent carbohydrates, 13 percent protein and 20 percent fat. On her light-workout days, her nutrient guidelines are 398 grams of carbohydrates, 57 grams of protein and 22 grams of fat for a total daily intake of 2,018 calories.

The menu below is for one of her hard-workout days. Please note that her actual intakes approximate her guidelines. There are days where she is slightly above her recommendations and others where she is slightly below, but on average she strives to come close to her desired intake levels. Also, Kimberly's menu is presented on a copy of the diet diary form (which you will find at the end of this chapter) to give you an example of how to complete the diary.

MEAL ITEMS	CARBOHYDRATES	PROTEIN	FAT	CALORIES
Breakfast: ½ cup nonfat granola, ½ cup oats, 1 cup applesauce, 1 cup calcium fortified low-fat milk	97 grams	18 grams	11 grams	530 calories
Lunch: Turkey sandwich on whole wheat bread, apple, carrots	83 grams	30 grams	19 grams	620 calories
Afternoon snack: medium banana 3 large, hard pretzels	96 grams	9 grams	0 grams	430 calories
Dinner: Salad w/ olive oil & vinegar, 12 oz. fish, large baked potato	88 grams	60 grams	26 grams	820 calories
Evening dessert: 1 cup whole fruit sorbet, 3 oz. mixed fruit	79 grams	0 grams	0 grams	300 calories
Pre Workout: Soy protein shake w/ rice milk	68 grams	8 grams	3 grams	330 calories
During run: Hydration drink	36 grams	0 grams	0 grams	140 calories
Post Workout: 1 energy bar	51 grams	7 grams	2 grams	250 calories
Daily Total:	*598 grams*	*132 grams*	*61 grams*	*3,420 calories*
Desired Daily Total:	*568 grams*	*114 grams*	*75 grams*	*3,403 calories*

MINIMUM of 8–10 glasses of water throughout day.

KIMBERLY'S DAILY DIET DIARY

MEAL	ITEMS	CALORIES (KCAL)	CARBOHYDRATE (G)	PROTEIN (G)	FAT (G)
Breakfast	½ cup nonfat granola, ½ cup oats, 1 cup applesauce, 1 cup calcium fortified low-fat milk	530	97	18	11
Snack					
Lunch	Turkey sandwich on whole wheat bread, apple, carrots	620	83	30	19
	SUB-TOTAL	1,150	180	48	30
Snack	medium banana 3 large, hard pretzels	430	96	9	0
Dinner	Salad w/ olive oil & vinegar, 12 oz. Fish, large baked potato, 1 cup whole fruit sorbet, 3 oz. mixed fruit	1,120	167	60	26

Exercise Intake:

TIME	PRODUCT(S)				
Before	Soy protein shake w/rice milk	330	68	8	3
During	Hydration drink	140	36	0	0
After	1 energy bar	250	51	7	2
	DAILY TOTAL	3,420	598	132	61
	DESIRED INTAKE	3,403	568	114	75

Kimberly has to work out right after she wakes up, and she has learned to eat before exercising. In the past, she would hit the trail without eating or drinking anything. As a result she was literally running on empty, was lethargic during the run, and famished later in the day. The solution was simple. By drinking a meal replacement shake immediately before heading out the door for her run, her energy levels were higher, her pace was faster, and her hunger was controllable.

Initially, she felt the *Fuel Up* program would be too much food for her to eat each day and that she would gain weight and get fat. After starting the diet, however, she was pleasantly surprised to find that she had actually lost a few pounds and that she was no longer lethargic and was no longer uncontrollably hungry later in the day.

Her boyfriend, Scott, is a thirty-six-year-old, 150-pound recreational athlete. He lifts weights four to five days a week and plays golf or tennis two to three days per week. He averages six workouts per week, two of which are hard weight workouts and one of which is an intense game of tennis. He wants to get leaner and more powerful, particularly in golf and tennis. Because he wants to lose weight he has limited his level of fat intake to 10 percent. On his hard-workout days his nutrient intake is 682 grams of carbohydrate, 136 grams of protein, and 40 grams of fat for a total daily caloric intake of 3,632 calories. On Scott's easy recovery-and-rest days he only needs 477 grams of carbohydrate, 68 grams of protein, and 27 grams of fat for a total daily intake of 2,423 calories. To satisfy these requirements, Scott enjoys menus like the following:

SAMPLE MENU FOR SCOTT'S HARD-WORKOUT DAYS:

	CALORIES (KCAL)	CARBOHYDRATE (G)	PROTEIN (G)	FAT (G)
Breakfast:				
2 slices toast	220	48	6	1
2 Tb. almond butter	220	6	8	18
2 Tb. 100% fruit jam	70	18	—	—
1 banana	100	24	1	—
1 c. nonfat milk	80	13	8	—
1 c. orange juice	105	24	—	—
	795	**133**	**23**	**19**
Snack:				
1⅓ c. oatmeal	300	54	15	6
¼ raisins	130	31	1	—
1 c. 100% fruit juice	140	35	—	—
	570	**120**	**16**	**6**
Lunch:				
1 can tuna	175	—	37	3
2 pickles, 1 tomato	50	11	—	—
2 slices bread	200	24	1	1
8 fat-free fig cookies	360	88	4	—
1 fruit juice nectar	190	54	—	—
	975	**177**	**42**	**4**
During Workout:				
4 c. hydration drink	200	56	—	—
Post Workout:				
1 energy bar	230	45	10	2.5
	430	**101**	**10**	**2.5**
Dinner:				
½ lb. fish	225	—	40	4
1½ c. steamed vegetables	75	19	—	—

	CALORIES (KCAL)	CARBOHYDRATE (G)	PROTEIN (G)	FAT (G)
2 c. rice	360	82	8	2
½ melon	100	24	—	—
2 c. vegetable juice	95	24	—	—
	855	149	48	6
Daily Total:	3,625	680	139	37.5
Desired Daily Total:	3,632	682	136	40

MINIMUM of 8–10 glasses of water throughout day.

SAMPLE MENU FOR SCOTT'S EASY-WORKOUT DAYS:

	CALORIES (KCAL)	CARBOHYDRATE (G)	PROTEIN (G)	FAT (G)
Breakfast:				
3 6-in. pancakes (made w/ nonfat milk & egg whites)	330	62	18	1
1 c. berries	60	14	1	—
1 c. applesauce	110	28	—	—
16 oz. orange juice	210	48	—	—
	710	152	19	1
Snack:				
30 g. pretzels	120	25	3	—
1 nectarine	100	24	1	—
	220	49	4	—
Lunch:				
1 large salad	205	36	4	1
balsamic vinegar & olive oil	120	—	—	14
2 slices bread	200	24	1	1
1 c. fruit juice nectar	190	54	—	—
	715	114	5	16

continued

	CALORIES (KCAL)	CARBOHYDRATE (G)	PROTEIN (G)	FAT (G)
During workout:				
2 c. Gatorade	100	28	—	—
	100	**28**	**—**	**—**
DINNER:				
4 oz. chicken	185	—	35	5
1 ear corn on the cob	95	21	3	1
1 baked potato	250	56	5	—
½ melon	100	24	—	—
1 c. vegetable juice	50	9	—	—
	680	**110**	**43**	**6**
Daily Total:	**2,425**	**453**	**71**	**23**
Desired Daily Total:	**2,423**	**477**	**68**	**27**

MINIMUM of 8–10 glasses of water throughout day.

An Athlete on the Go: No Time to Eat

Scott and Kimberly's friend George is a 53-year-old, 175-pound athlete who is typical of today's business executive. He routinely puts in 12-hour days, 6 days a week, and has no time to cook. Unable to sit down and eat meals for breakfast or lunch, he has given up fast food and relies on meal replacement shakes, bars, and protein supplements to provide his diet with the necessary nutrients. He has sacrificed taste for function, but couldn't be happier thanks to the improvement he's seen in his performance.

SAMPLE MENU FOR PEOPLE ON THE GO:

	CALORIES (KCAL)	CARBOHYDRATE (G)	PROTEIN (G)	FAT (G)
Breakfast:				
1 scoop protein	110	2	25	—
1 c. orange juice	105	24	—	—
1 c. frozen berries	60	14	1	—
1 bagel	250	56	3	1
	525	**96**	**29**	**1**
Snack:				
16 oz. smoothie	320	64	2	9
1 c. applesauce	110	28	—	—
⅔ c. oats	200	36	10	4
¼ c. raisins	130	31	1	—
	760	**159**	**13**	**13**
Lunch:				
1 meal replacement bar	190	24	14	4
2 pieces fruit	200	48	2	—
	390	**72**	**16**	**4**
During workout:				
3 c. Gatorade	150	42	—	—
	150	**42**	**—**	**—**
Dinner:				
1 large spaghetti & sauce	305	36	16	6
1½ c. steamed vegetables	75	19	—	—
3 slices Italian bread	310	64	9	1
1 c. sorbet	240	70	—	—
	930	**189**	**25**	**7**
Daily Total:	**2,755**	**558**	**83**	**25**
Desired Daily Total:	**2,839**	**560**	**80**	**31**

MINIMUM of 8–10 glasses of water throughout day.

The Three Stages of Sports Nutrition: When Is As Important As What

The second component of *Fuel Up* involves timing: Knowing when to eat the nutrients you need is as important as knowing what to eat. We will see that supplying your body with adequate energy has three different sets of guidelines for: before, during, and after the workout or activity.

Before Exercise

The purpose of a preworkout meal is the provision of adequate carbohydrates and fluid. When deciding what to eat, pay special attention to the foods' digestibility. As a rule, avoid foods high in fat and protein because these foods are digested slowly and remain in the digestive tract longer than carbohydrates. If you have been under a lot of stress or are in a race, the extra tension will decrease blood flow to the digestive tract and decrease intestinal absorption.

To improve performance, eat between 150 to 300 grams of carbo-hydrates in a meal 3 to 4 hours before the workout. This guarantees maximal liver and muscle glycogen stores, which maximize your muscle power and performance.

Eating anything, particularly food with a high glycemic index, within the hour before exercise can impair performance. The ele-vated blood sugar levels cause an excess release of insulin into the bloodstream. These high insulin levels inhibit fat breakdown from adipose tissue and produce a greater reliance on carbohydrate stores. In turn, this causes inordinately large increases in carbohydrate metabolism, rapid muscle glycogen depletion, and early fatigue. For that reason, don't eat less than 60 minutes before an event.

If you don't have time to eat more than an hour before the workout, hold off until you start warming up. Limit the fluid you drink within the hour prior to your exercise to water. Drinking a meal replacement shake minutes before the actual exercise begins is a good alternative because these meals are high in carbohydrates, supply fuel immediately, and leave no residue in the intestinal tract. Because they are liquid, they also contribute to your fluid requirements. In addition, they are particularly effective during day-long events such as century bike rides, long hikes, and tennis, soccer, or basketball tournaments. Also, drinking them immediately after a match or heat will give sufficient time for digestion and absorption to take place before you begin again.

During Exercise

An hour-long, high-intensity aerobic workout can decrease liver glycogen by 55 percent. A two-hour workout almost completely depletes the glycogen content of the liver and muscles used in the activity. Repetitive activities such as weight lifting, ice hockey, and football when performed at maximal levels can dramatically lower liver and muscle glycogen reserves in very short periods of time.

Supplying carbohydrates during exercise helps maintain blood glucose stores and tempers liver and muscle glycogen breakdown. Scientific studies conclusively show that liquid or solid carbohydrates consumed during exercise significantly improve performance in high-intensity, long-term aerobic exercise and repetitive short bouts of near-maximal effort. Even at moderate intensity levels (60–80 percent of maximal aerobic capacity), fatigue is postponed by 15 to 30 minutes with carbohydrate feeding during exercise.

Drinking 8 ounces of a hydration beverage containing 6 to 8 percent carbohydrates every 15 minutes helps maintain adequate blood glucose to supply energy and to maintain optimal hydration. You can get the same effect by eating a piece of fruit or an energy bar and drinking one to two cups of water. Remember that your thirst is a poor indicator of your hydration level, particularly during exercise. Even if you think you don't need to, make sure you get enough to drink.

After Exercise

The most important nutrient to replace after the workout is water. Since exercise dulls thirst, you must again make a conscious effort to replace the lost fluids. Besides following the hydration guidelines, the most accurate way to gauge how much fluid you need is by weighing yourself without clothing before and after the exercise. Drink two cups of fluid for every pound you lost. If you have to perform another round of exercise relatively soon thereafter, such as in a tournament, you might require as much as three cups per pound of weight lost to achieve rehydration.

In addition to water, you should begin carbohydrate replacement as soon after training or competition as possible. When you delay consumption of carbohydrates, the rate of glycogen synthesis is almost half of that when carbohydrates are consumed within the first one to two hours after exercise.

Current recommendations suggest ingesting 0.5 grams of carbohydrate per pound of body weight immediately after exercise. Follow that by eating 50 to 75 grams of carbohydrates with high to moderate glycemic levels every hour until you've consumed 500 grams. More rapid resynthesis also takes place if you are inactive during the recovery period. With optimal carbohydrate intake, glycogen is restored at rates of 5 to 7 percent per hour. Under the best circumstances, it still takes at least 20 hours after a glycogen-depleting workout to return to pre-exercise glycogen levels.

Protein intake during the postexercise phase is also extremely important. Mark Tarnopolsky, Ph.D., has shown that the recommended dose of carbohydrates immediately after and then 60 minutes after resistance exercise also helps protein metabolism by decreasing protein breakdown and enhancing retention of muscle protein stores. Further studies by John Ivy, Ph.D., et al., and others have shown that combining protein with carbohydrates in the post-exercise meal increases glycogen synthesis. Consequently eating protein at a level set at 20 to 40 percent of the carbohydrate intake immediately after the exercise, as well as 60 and 120 minutes afterward, will enhance glycogen repletion and recovery.

Eating protein immediately after also plays a role in tissue repair and growth. Researchers theorize that postexercise protein shortens recovery and stimulates muscle development. In a 1997 study, Robert Wolfe, Ph.D., et al. showed that the availability of free amino acids immediately after exercise increases muscle anabolism by increasing protein synthesis and decreasing protein breakdown.

Protein intake appears to be particularly important in exercise that results in muscle damage such as repetitive power workouts to exhaustion, intense endurance exercise, eccentric exercise (that produces force during muscle lengthening), two workouts a day, and contact sports.

Eating or drinking foods with a combination of 50 to 75 grams of carbohydrate and 10 to 30 grams of protein immediately after exercise and for the first few hours thereafter is essential. Once you're ready to sit down and eat, plan your meal to reflect a wider range of required nutrients, including fat.

Although the timing of what you eat is critical to your performance, it is not a miracle cure. One meal cannot correct long-term nutritional inadequacies. True sports nutrition has to be practiced throughout training, in the weeks and months prior to any competition or event, not just several days before.

The Performance of Your Life

Now, at last, you have the whole picture. You've got the principles of sports nutrition and the tools to personalize them. I have. After a lifetime of competition, I can tell you that by following these principles, my performance has improved to levels that are surprising to myself, my teammates, and my competitors. My training has never been so consistent or free of setbacks. My attitude is more positive, knowing that my training and diet are based upon state-of-the-art science. And I have never had as much fun. Now it's your turn. Enjoy!

Hydration Diary

MAINTENANCE H$_2$O:

	1	2	3	4	5	6	7	8	9	10
yes / 1 cup										

Place a check in each box for each cup of water you drink throughout the day to meet the 8-to-10-cup-per-day maintenance guideline.

EXERCISE HYDRATION:

PRIOR

(2 hours before)

	1	2	3
yes / 1 cup			

(15 minutes before)

	1	2	3
yes / 1 cup			

DURING

(Every 15–20 minutes)

	1	2	3	4	5	6	7	8
yes / 1 cup								

229

AFTER

Pre-exercise weight:_____ lbs. / Postexercise weight:_____ lbs.
Exercise weight loss:_____ lbs.

(Every 30 minutes)

	1	2	3	4	5	6	7	8
yes / 1 cup								

Place a check in each box for each cup you drink after exercise. For optimal fluid and carbohydrate intake, drink **two cups** every 30 minutes post exercise for each **one** pound of weight lost during exercise.

NUTRIENT INTAKE DURING DAILY FLUID HYDRATION:

CALORIES	PROTEIN	CARBOHYDRATE	TOTAL FAT
Cal/day	grams/day	grams/day	grams/day

It is important to remember not to restrict fluid intake before, during, or after exercise. Avoid beverages containing caffeine, alcohol, or other diuretic agents because they increase urine production and add to dehydration.

Daily Diet Diary

MEAL	ITEMS	CALORIES (KCAL)	CARBOHYDRATE (G)	PROTEIN (G)	FAT (G)
Breakfast					
Snack					
Lunch					
SUBTOTAL					
Snack					

MEAL	ITEMS	CALORIES (KCAL)	CARBOHYDRATE (G)	PROTEIN (G)	FAT (G)
Dinner					
Exercise Intake: TIME PRODUCT(S)					
Before					
During					
After					
DAILY TOTAL					
DESIRED INTAKE					

*Total fat level (10 or 20%) can be selected based on your current dietary intake and overall health goals.

Nutritive Values for Selected Foods

The appendix lists the nutritive values for selected common foods. The foods are broken down into carbohydrate and protein sources and sorted by food category and content. The serving size, caloric content, and amount of carbohydrate, protein, and fat are listed for each food. The foods grouped in categories are listed based on content of either carbohydrate or protein.

CARBOHYDRATE CONTENT

Sorted by category

FOOD	CARBOHYDRATE	CALORIES	PROTEIN	FAT	SERVING SIZE
Carbonated Beverages					
Mountain Dew	44.4	179	0	0	12 oz
Coke	40.0	154	0	0	12 oz
Pepsi-Cola	39.6	160	0	0	12 oz
Root Beer	39.2	152	0	0	12 oz
Coke Classic	38.0	144	0	0	12 oz
Dr Pepper	37.2	144	0	0	12 oz

continued 233

FOOD	CARBOHYDRATE	CALORIES	PROTEIN	FAT	SERVING SIZE
7UP	36.2	144	0	0	12 oz
Lemon Lime	36.0	142	0	0	12 oz
Sprite	36.0	142	0	0	12 oz
Ginger Ale	31.9	124	0	0	12 oz
Fruit Juice Drinks & Fruit Flavored Beverages					
Cranberry Apple Drink	41.9	164	0	0	8 oz
Cranberry Drink	36.5	144	0	0	8 oz
Grape Drink	32.3	125	0	0	8 oz
Kool-Aid	25.1	98	0	0	8 oz
Cereals, Cooked or to be Cooked					
Barley, Pearled	44.3	193	3.6	0.7	1 Cup
Couscous	41.6	201	6.8	0.0	1 Cup
Cream of Rice	29.7	143	4.1	0.5	1 Cup
Bran Rasin Quaker	29.2	153	5.2	1.7	¾ Cooked
Raisins, Dates & Walnuts	25.1	141	4.0	3.8	1.3 oz Dry
Total	22.0	110	4.0	2.0	1.2 oz Dry
Malt-O-Meal	21.1	100	3.6	0.4	1 Cup
Oatmeal, Quick	18.6	99	4.4	2.0	⅔ Cooked
Cereals, Ready to Eat					
Grape-Nuts	92.4	420	12.4	0.4	1 Cup
100% Natural	72.0	508	13.2	22.0	1 Cup
All-Bran	66.0	210	12	3.0	1 Cup
Corn Flakes	58.2	220	7.8	12.3	1 Cup
Fiber One	46.0	120	4.0	2.0	1 Cup
Fruit & Fibre	43.4	182	5.6	2.0	1 Cup
Apple Raisin	42.6	173	2.6	0.0	1 Cup
Clusters	40.0	220	6.0	6.0	1 Cup
Corn Bran	31.0	145	2.9	1.2	1 Cup
Bran Chex	30.6	120	3.8	0.9	1 Cup
Oat Bran	25.0	125	6.2	2.5	1 Cup
Rice Krispies	24.8	110	1.9	0.2	1 Cup
Cheerios	15.6	88	3.4	1.4	1 Cup
Cheese & Cheese Products					
Ricotta, Skim	6.4	171	14.1	9.8	½ Cup
Ricotta, Whole	3.8	216	14	16.1	½ Cup
Cottage Cheese, 1%	3.1	82	14	1.1	4 oz

FOOD	CARBOHYDRATE	CALORIES	PROTEIN	FAT	SERVING SIZE
Cottage Cheese	3.0	117	14.1	5.1	4 oz
Cream Cheese, Light	1.8	62	2.9	4.7	1 oz
Feta	1.2	75	4.0	6.0	1 oz
Cheddar, Extra Sharp	1.0	100	6.0	9.0	1 oz
Swiss	1.0	107	8.1	7.8	1 oz
Chips, Pretzels, Popcorn & Similar Snack Foods					
Pretzels	22.5	108	2.6	1.0	1 oz
Keebler Pretzels	21.0	104	2.8	0.8	1 oz
French Onion Light	19.0	134	2.0	5.9	1 oz
Air-Popped Popcorn	18.9	92.5	2.9	1.0	3 Cups
Trail Mix Tropical	18.6	115	1.8	4.9	1 oz
Chex Mix	18.5	121	3.1	4.9	1 oz
Tortilla Chips	17.8	142	2.0	7.4	1 oz
Banana Chips	16.6	147	0.7	9.5	1 oz
Potato Sticks	15.1	148	1.9	9.8	1 oz
Barbecue Chips	15.0	139	2.2	9.2	1 oz
French Onion	13.0	170	2.0	11.0	1 oz
Trail Mix	12.7	131	3.9	8.3	1 oz
Microwave Popcorn with butter	10.0	90	2.0	6.0	3 Cups
Fast Foods					
Burrito with Beef	58.5	523	26.6	20.8	2 Burritos
Chocolate Shake	57.9	360	9.6	10.5	10 oz
Burrito with Bean & Cheese	55.0	337	15.1	11.7	2 Burritos
Vanilla Shake	50.8	314	9.8	8.4	10 oz
French Toast Sticks	49.1	479	8.3	29.1	5 Sticks
Cheeseburger, Large	47.4	608	30.1	33.0	1 Sandwich
Baked Potato with Cheese	46.5	475	14.6	28.7	1 Potato
French Fries	44.4	355	4.6	18.5	Large Order
Chicken Fillet	38.7	515	24.1	29.5	1 Sandwich
Corn on the Cob with butter	32.0	155	4.5	3.4	1 Ear
Onion Rings	31.3	275	3.7	15.5	8–9 Rings
Biscuit with Egg & Ham	30.3	442	20.4	27.0	1 Biscuit
English Muffin with butter	30.3	189	4.9	5.8	1 Muffin
French Fries	29.3	235	3.0	12.2	Reg Order
Bacon Cheeseburger	29.1	464	25.1	27.3	1 Sandwich
Danish Pastry, Cheese	28.7	353	5.8	24.6	3.2 oz Pastry
Fried Chicken with Honey	26.9	329	16.8	17.5	6 Pieces

continued

FOOD	CARBOHYDRATE	CALORIES	PROTEIN	FAT	SERVING SIZE
Cheeseburger, Regular	26.5	295	16	14.1	1 Sandwich
Croissant with Egg & Cheese	24.3	369	12.8	24.7	1 Croissant
Biscuit with Egg	24.2	315	11.1	20.2	1 Biscuit
Chicken, Breaded, Fried	15.5	290	16.9	17.7	6 Pieces
Crab Cake	5.1	160	11.3	10.4	2.1 oz Cake
Fruit & Vegetable Juices					
Peach Nectar	34.7	134	0.7	0.0	8 oz
Pineapple Juice	34.4	139	0.8	0.0	8 oz
Apple Juice	29.0	116	0.0	0.0	8 oz
Orange Juice	24.5	104	1.5	0.4	8 oz
Carrot Juice	22.8	97	2.2	0.4	8 oz
Grapefruit Juice	22.7	96	1.2	0.3	8 oz
Tomato Juice	10.9	43	1.8	0.2	8 oz
Fruits					
Dates, Dried	61.0	228	1.6	0.4	10 Dates
Applesauce, sweetened	51.0	194	0.4	0.4	1 Cup
Mango, Raw	35.2	135	1.1	0.6	1 Medium
Papaya, Raw	29.8	117	1.9	0.4	1 Medium
Applesauce, Can	28.0	114	0.0	0.0	1 Cup
Banana, Raw	26.7	105	1.2	0.6	1 Medium
Pear	25.1	98	0.7	0.7	1 Medium
Apple, Raw	21.1	81	0.0	0.5	1 Medium
Blueberries, Raw	20.5	82	1.0	0.6	1 Cup
Pineapple, Raw	19.2	77	0.6	0.7	1 Cup
Apple Raw, No Skin	19.0	72	0.0	0.4	1 Medium
Blackberries, Raw	18.4	74	1.0	0.6	1 Cup
Orange	16.3	65	1.4	0.0	1 Medium
Honeydew Melon, Raw	15.6	60	0.8	0.0	1 Cup
Raspberries, Raw	14.2	61	1.1	0.7	1 Cup
Cantaloupe, Raw	13.4	57	1.4	0.4	1 Cup
Raisins, Seedless	13.0	50	0.5	0.0	⅛ Cup
Watermelon, Raw	11.5	50	1.0	0.7	1 Cup
Kiwifruit, Raw	11.3	46	0.8	0.0	1 Medium
Cherries Sweet, Raw	11.3	49	0.8	0.7	10 Cherries
Guava, Raw	10.7	45	0.7	0.5	1 Medium
Strawberries, Raw	10.5	45	0.9	0.6	1 Cup
Peach, Raw	9.7	37	0.6	0.0	1 Medium

FOOD	CARBOHYDRATE	CALORIES	PROTEIN	FAT	SERVING SIZE
Figs, Raw	9.6	37	0.4	0.0	1 Medium
Grapefruit, Raw	9.5	37	0.7	0.0	1 Medium
Tangerine, Raw	9.4	37	0.5	0.0	1 Cup
Plum, Raw	8.6	36	0.5	0.4	1 Medium
Avocado, Raw	6.0	153	1.8	15.0	½ Medium
Breads, Yeast					
Bagel	30.9	163	6.0	1.4	1 Bagel
Pita Bread/Pocket	20.6	106	4.0	0.6	1 Pocket
Pumpernickel	15.4	82	2.9	0.8	1 Slice
Raisin	13.2	70	2.1	1.0	1 Slice
Oatmeal	13.0	71	2.4	1.2	1 Slice
Honey & Oat Bran	12.7	71	3.2	1.2	1 Slice
Cracked Wheat	12.5	66	2.3	0.9	1 Slice
Rye	12.0	66	2.1	0.9	1 Slice
White	11.7	64	2.0	0.9	1 Slice
Whole Wheat	11.4	61	2.4	1.1	1 Slice
Wheat	11.3	61	2.3	1.0	1 Slice
Stone ground	9.9	48	2.4	0.7	1 Slice
Crackers					
Breadflats	10.6	53	1.3	0.8	1 Slice
Triscuits	10.0	60	1.0	2.0	3 Crackers
Cheese Nips	9.0	70	1.0	3.0	13 Crackers
Ritz	9.0	70	1.0	4.0	4 Crackers
Wheat Thins	9.0	70	1.0	3.0	8 Crackers
Chicken in a Biskit	8.0	80	1.0	5.0	7 Crackers
Zwieback	5.2	30	0.7	0.6	1 Piece
Crispbread	5.0	25	1.0	0.0	1 Piece
Saltines	4.4	26	0.6	0.6	2 Crackers
Club	4.2	34	0.5	1.4	2 Crackers
Muffins					
English Muffin	26.2	135	4.5	1.1	1 Muffin
Corn	20.0	130	2.8	4.2	1 Muffin
Raisin Bran	16.8	121	2.7	4.8	1 Muffin
Bran	16.7	112	3.0	5.1	1 Muffin
Pasta					
Fettuccine, Spinach	65.0	360	17.0	5.0	4.5 oz
Macaroni, Enriched	39.7	197	6.7	0.9	1 Cup

continued

FOOD	CARBOHYDRATE	CALORIES	PROTEIN	FAT	SERVING SIZE
Macaroni, Wheat	37.2	174	7.5	0.8	1 Cup
Egg Noodles	30.5	166	4.5	1.0	4.5 oz
Chow Mein	25.9	237	3.8	13.8	1 Cup
Japanese Soba	24.4	113	5.8	0.0	1 Cup
Milk, Yogurt, Milk Beverages & Milk Beverage Mixes					
Buttermilk, Cultured	11.7	99	8.1	2.2	8 oz
Low Fat, 1%	11.7	102	8.0	2.6	8 oz
Skim	11.9	86	8.4	0.4	8 oz
Goat	10.9	168	8.7	10.1	8 oz
Soy	4.3	79	6.6	4.6	8oz
Vanilla Yogurt	37.2	200	10.6	0.0	8 oz
Yogurt, Skim with Fruit	38.2	200	10.1	0.0	8 oz
Yogurt, Skim	17.4	127	13.0	0.4	8 oz
Sauces, Condiments & Gravies					
Spaghetti Sauce, Can	20.0	136	2.2	6.0	½ Cup
Marinara Sauce	12.7	86	2.0	4.2	½ Cup
Salsa	12.0	50	2.0	0.0	3 oz
Pesto Sauce	9.0	465	8.4	43.8	3 oz
Contadina Fresh	5.0	270	4.5	26.5	3 oz
Ketchup	4.1	16	0.0	0.0	1 T
Teriyaki Sauce	2.9	15	1.1	0.0	1 T
Horseradish Sauce	2.3	54	0.0	4.9	1 T
Barbeque Sauce	2.0	12	0.0	0.3	1 T
Soups					
Tomato	40.3	208	5.0	4.7	1 Can
Black Bean	34.0	206	10.6	3.0	1 Cup
Green Pea	26.5	164	8.6	2.9	1 Cup
Beef Broth	24.7	130	5.5	1.0	1 Cup
Cream of Mushroom	22.6	313	4.9	23.1	1 Can
Cream of Chicken	22.5	283	8.3	17.9	1 Can
Black Bean	19.8	116	5.6	1.5	1 Cup
Clam Chowder	12.2	77	2.2	2.2	1 Cup
Minestrone	11.2	83	4.3	2.5	1 Cup
Cream of Asparagus	10.4	81	2.1	3.5	1 Cup
Chicken Noodle	9.4	75	4.0	2.5	1 Cup
Chicken Vegetable	8.6	74	3.6	2.8	1 Cup
Turkey Noodle	8.6	69	3.9	2.0	1 Cup

FOOD	CARBOHYDRATE	CALORIES	PROTEIN	FAT	SERVING SIZE
Onion	8.2	57	3.8	1.7	1 Cup
Chicken Broth	0.9	39	4.9	1.4	1 Cup
Vegetables, Vegetable Products & Vegetable Salads					
Baked Beans	27.5	191	7.0	6.5	½ Cup
Hummus	24.8	210	6.5	10.4	½ Cup
Refried Beans	23.4	135	7.9	1.3	½ Cup
White Corn	21.5	100	2.4	0.4	½ Cup
Yellow Corn	20.6	89	2.7	1.1	½ Cup
Kidney Beans	20.2	112	7.7	0.4	½ Cup
Lima Beans	19.7	108	7.3	0.0	½ Cup
Artichoke	13.4	60	4.2	0.0	1 Medium
Artichoke Heart	8.7	37	1.9	0.0	½ Cup
Leeks	7.4	32	0.8	0.0	½ Cup
Carrots	7.3	31	0.7	0.0	1 Medium
Brussels Sprouts	6.8	30	2.0	0.4	½ Cup
Pumpkin	6.0	24	0.9	0.0	½ Cup
Tomato	5.7	26	1.0	0.4	1 Tomato
Tofu	5.4	183	19.9	11.0	½ Cup
Green Beans	4.9	22	1.2	0.0	½ Cup
Broccoli	2.3	12	1.3	0.0	½ Cup
Red Cabbage	2.1	10	0.5	0.0	½ Cup
Green Cabbage	1.9	8	0.4	0.0	½ Cup
Mushrooms	1.6	9	0.7	0.0	½ Cup
Garlic	1.0	4	0.0	0.0	1 Clove
Carbohydrate Content: Sorted by amount					
Grape-Nuts	92.4	420	12.4	0.4	1 Cup
100% Natural Granola	72.0	508	13.2	22.0	1 Cup
All-Bran	66.0	210	12.0	3.0	1 Cup
Fettuccine, Spinach	65.0	360	17.0	5.0	4.5 oz
Dates, Dried	61.0	228	1.6	0.4	10 Dates
Burrito with Beef	58.5	523	26.6	20.8	2 Burritos
Corn Flakes	58.2	220	7.8	12.3	1 Cup
Chocolate Shake	57.9	360	9.6	10.5	10 oz
Burrito with Bean & Cheese	55.0	337	15.1	11.7	2 Burritos
Applesauce, Sweetened	51.0	194	0.4	0.4	1 Cup
Vanilla Shake	50.8	314	9.8	8.4	10 oz
French Toast Sticks	49.1	479	8.3	29.1	5 Sticks

continued

FOOD	CARBOHYDRATE	CALORIES	PROTEIN	FAT	SERVING SIZE
Cheeseburger, Large	47.4	608	30.1	33.0	1 Sandwich
Baked Potato with Cheese	46.5	475	14.6	28.7	1 Potato
Fiber One	46.0	120	4.0	2.0	1 Cup
French Fries	44.4	355	4.6	18.5	Large Order
Mountain Dew	44.4	179	0.0	0.0	12 oz
Barley, Pearled	44.3	193	3.6	0.7	1 Cup
Fruit & Fibre Cereal	43.4	182	5.6	2.0	1 Cup
Apple Raisin	42.6	173	2.6	0.0	1 Cup
Cranberry Apple Drink	41.9	164	0.0	0.0	8 oz
Couscous	41.6	201	6.8	0.0	1 Cup
Tomato Soup	40.3	208	5.0	4.7	1 Can
Clusters Cereal	40.0	220	6.0	6.0	1 Cup
Coke	40.0	154	0.0	0.0	12 oz
Macaroni, Enriched	39.7	197	6.7	0.9	1 Cup
Pepsi Cola	39.6	160	0.0	0.0	12 oz
Root Beer	39.2	152	0.0	0.0	12 oz
Chicken Fillet	38.7	515	24.1	29.5	1 Sandwich
Yogurt, Skim with Fruit	38.2	200	10.1	0.0	8 oz
Coke Classic	38.0	144	0.0	0.0	12 oz
Vanilla Yogurt	37.2	200	10.6	0.0	8 oz
Macaroni, Wheat	37.2	174	7.5	0.8	1 Cup
Dr Pepper	37.2	144	0.0	0.0	12 oz
Cranberry Drink	36.5	144	0.0	0.0	8 oz
7UP	36.2	144	0.0	0.0	12 oz
Lemon Lime	36.0	142	0.0	0.0	12 oz
Sprite	36.0	142	0.0	0.0	12 oz
Mango, Raw	35.2	135	1.1	0.6	1 Medium
Peach Nectar	34.7	134	0.7	0.0	8 oz
Pineapple Juice	34.4	139	0.8	0.0	8 oz
Black Bean Soup	34.0	206	10.6	3.0	1 Cup
Grape Drink	32.3	125	0.0	0.0	8 oz
Corn on the Cob with butter	32.0	155	4.5	3.4	1 Ear
Ginger Ale	31.9	124	0.0	0.0	12 oz
Onion Rings	31.3	275	3.7	15.5	8-9 Rings
Corn Bran	31.0	145	2.9	1.2	1 Cup
Bagel	30.9	163	6.0	1.4	1 Bagel
Bran Chex	30.6	120	3.8	0.9	1 Cup
Egg Noodles	30.5	166	4.5	1.0	4.5 oz

FOOD	CARBOHYDRATE	CALORIES	PROTEIN	FAT	SERVING SIZE
Biscuit with Egg & Ham	30.3	442	20.4	27.0	1 Biscuit
English Muffin with butter	30.3	189	4.9	5.8	1 Muffin
Papaya, Raw	29.8	117	1.9	0.4	1 Medium
Cream of Rice	29.7	143	4.1	0.5	1 Cup
French Fries	29.3	235	3.0	12.2	Reg Order
Bran Raisin Quaker	29.2	153	5.2	1.7	¾ Cooked
Bacon Cheeseburger	29.1	464	25.1	27.3	1 Sandwich
Apple Juice	29.0	116	0.0	0.0	8 oz
Danish Pastry, Cheese	28.7	353	5.8	24.6	3.2oz Pastry
Applesauce, Can	28.0	114	0.0	0.0	1 Cup
Baked Beans	27.5	191	7.0	6.5	½ Cup
Fried Chicken with Honey	26.9	329	16.8	17.5	6 Pieces
Banana, Raw	26.7	105	1.2	0.6	1 Medium
Cheeseburger, Regular	26.5	295	16.0	14.1	1 Sandwich
Green Pea Soup	26.5	164	8.6	2.9	1 Cup
English Muffin	26.2	135	4.5	1.1	1 Muffin
Chow Mein	25.9	237	3.8	13.8	1 Cup
Raisins, Dates, & Walnuts	25.1	141	4.0	3.8	1.3oz Dry
Pear	25.1	98	0.7	0.7	1 Medium
Kool-Aid	25.1	98	0.0	0.0	8 oz
Oat Bran	25.0	125	6.2	2.5	1 Cup
Hummus	24.8	210	6.5	10.4	½ Cup
Rice Krispies	24.8	110	1.9	0.0	1 Cup
Beef Broth	24.7	130	5.5	1.0	1 Cup
Orange Juice	24.5	104	1.5	0.4	8 oz
Japanese Soba	24.4	113	5.8	0.1	1 Cup
Croissant with Egg &Cheese	24.3	369	12.8	24.7	1 Croissant
Biscuit with Egg	24.2	315	11.1	20.2	1 Biscuit
Refried Beans	23.4	135	7.9	1.3	½ Cup
Carrot Juice	22.8	97	2.2	0.4	8 oz
Grapefruit Juice	22.7	96	1.2	0.0	8 oz
Cream of Mushroom Soup	22.6	313	4.9	23.1	1 Can
Cream of Chicken Soup	22.5	283	8.3	17.9	1 Can
Pretzels	22.5	108	2.6	1.0	1 oz
Total	22.0	110	4.0	2.0	1.2oz Dry
White Corn	21.5	100	2.4	0.4	½ Cup
Malt-O-Meal	21.1	100	3.6	0.4	1 Cup
Apple, Raw	21.1	81	0.0	0.5	1 Medium

continued

FOOD	CARBOHYDRATE	CALORIES	PROTEIN	FAT	SERVING SIZE
Keebler Pretzels	21.0	104	2.8	0.8	1oz
Pita Bread/pocket	20.6	106	4.0	0.6	1 Pocket
Yellow Corn	20.6	89	2.7	1.1	½ Cup
Blueberries, Raw	20.5	82	1.0	0.6	1 Cup
Kidney Beans	20.2	112	7.7	0.4	½ Cup
Spaghetti Sauce, Can	20.0	136	2.2	6.0	½ Cup
Corn Muffin	20.0	130	2.8	4.2	1 Muffin
Lima Beans	19.7	108	7.3	0.3	½ Cup
Pineapple, Raw	19.2	77	0.6	0.7	1 Cup
French Onion Light	19.0	134	2.0	5.9	1oz
Apple, Raw, No Skin	19.0	72	0.0	0.4	1 Medium
Air-Popped Corn	18.9	92.5	2.9	1.0	3 Cups
Oatmeal, Quick	18.6	99	4.4	2.0	⅔ Cooked
Trail Mix, Tropical	18.6	115	1.8	4.9	1oz
Chex Mix	18.5	121	3.1	4.9	1oz
Blackberries, Raw	18.4	74	1.0	0.6	1 Cup
Tortilla Chips	17.8	142	2.0	7.4	1oz
Yogurt, Skim	17.4	127	13	0.4	8oz
Raisin Bran	16.8	121	2.7	4.8	1 Muffin
Bran Muffin	16.7	112	3.0	5.1	1 Muffin
Banana Chips	16.6	147	0.7	9.5	1oz
Orange	16.3	65	1.4	0.1	1 Medium
Cheerios	15.6	88	3.4	1.4	1 Cup
Honeydew Melon, Raw	15.6	60	0.8	0.2	1 Cup
Chicken, Breaded, Fried	15.5	290	16.9	17.7	6 Pieces
Pumpernickel Bread	15.4	82	2.9	0.8	1 Slice
Potato Sticks	15.1	148	1.9	9.8	1oz
Barbecue Chips	15.0	139	2.2	9.2	1oz
Raspberries, Raw	14.2	61	1.1	0.7	1 Cup
Artichoke	13.4	60	4.2	0.0	1 Medium
Cantaloupe, Raw	13.4	57	1.4	0.4	1 Cup
Raisin Bread	13.2	70	2.1	1.0	1 Slice
Raisins, Seedless	13.0	50	0.5	0.0	⅛ Cup
Oatmeal Bread	13.0	71	2.4	1.2	1 Slice
French Onion Chips	13.0	170	2.0	11.0	1oz
Marinara Sauce	12.7	86	2.0	4.2	½ Cup
Trail Mix	12.7	131	3.9	8.3	1oz
Honey & Oat Bran Bread	12.7	71	3.2	1.2	1 Slice

FOOD	CARBOHYDRATE	CALORIES	PROTEIN	FAT	SERVING SIZE
Cracked Wheat Bread	12.5	66	2.3	0.9	1 Slice
Clam Chowder	12.2	77	2.2	2.2	1 Cup
Rye Bread	12.0	66	2.1	0.9	1 Slice
Salsa	12.0	50	2.0	0.0	3 oz
Skim Milk	11.9	86	8.4	0.4	8oz
Buttermilk, Cultured	11.7	99	8.1	2.2	8oz
Low-fat Milk, 1%	11.7	102	8.0	2.6	8oz
White Bread	11.7	64	2.0	0.9	1 Slice
Watermelon, Raw	11.5	50	1.0	0.7	1 Cup
Whole Wheat Bread	11.4	61	2.4	1.1	1 Slice
Wheat Bread	11.3	61	2.3	1.0	1 Slice
Kiwifruit, Raw	11.3	46	0.8	0.0	1 Medium
Cherries, Sweet, Raw	11.3	49	0.8	0.7	10 Cherries
Minestrone	11.2	83	4.3	2.5	1 Cup
Goat Milk	10.9	168	8.7	10.1	8oz
Tomato Juice	10.9	43	1.8	0.0	8oz
Guava, Raw	10.7	45	0.7	0.5	1 Medium
Breadflats	10.6	53	1.3	0.8	1 Slice
Strawberries, Raw	10.5	45	0.9	0.6	1 Cup
Cream of Asparagus Soup	10.4	81	2.1	3.5	1 Cup
Microwave Popcorn with butter	10.0	90	2.0	6.0	3 Cups
Triscuits	10.0	60	1.0	2.0	3 Crackers
Stone Ground Bread	9.9	48	2.4	0.7	1 Slice
Peach, Raw	9.7	37	0.6	0.0	1 Medium
Figs, Raw	9.6	37	0.4	0.0	1 Medium
Grapefruit, Raw	9.5	37	0.7	0.0	1 Medium
Chicken Noodle Soup	9.4	75	4.0	2.5	1 Cup
Tangerine, Raw	9.4	37	0.5	0.0	1 Cup
Pesto Sauce	9.0	465	8.4	43.8	3oz
Cheese Nips	9.0	70	1.0	3.0	13 Crackers
Ritz	9.0	70	1.0	4.0	4 Crackers
Wheat Thins	9.0	70	1.0	3.0	8 Crackers
Artichoke Heart	8.7	37	1.9	0.0	½ Cup
Turkey Noodle Soup	8.6	69	3.9	2.0	1 Cup
Chicken Vegetable Soup	8.6	74	3.6	2.8	1 Cup
Plum, Raw	8.6	36	0.5	0.4	1 Medium
Onion Soup	8.2	57	3.8	1.7	1 Cup
Chicken in a Biskit	8.0	80	1.0	5.0	7 Crackers

continued

FOOD	CARBOHYDRATE	CALORIES	PROTEIN	FAT	SERVING SIZE
Leeks	7.4	32	0.8	0.0	½ Cup
Carrots	7.3	31	0.7	0.0	1 Medium
Lime, Raw	7.1	20	0.5	0.0	1 Medium
Brussels Sprouts	6.8	30	2.0	0.4	½ Cup
Ricotta, Skim	6.4	171	14.1	9.8	½ Cup
Avocado, Raw	6.0	153	1.8	15.0	½ Medium
Pumpkin	6.0	24	0.9	0.0	½ Cup
Tomato	5.7	26	1.0	0.4	1 Tomato
Tofu	5.4	183	19.9	11.0	½ Cup
Lemon, Raw	5.4	17	0.6	0.0	1 Medium
Zwieback	5.2	30	0.7	0.6	1 Piece
Crab Cake	5.1	160	11.3	10.4	2.1oz Cake
Contadina, Fresh	5.0	270	4.5	26.5	3oz
Crispbread	5.0	25	1.0	0.0	1 Piece
Green Beans	4.9	22	1.2	0.0	½ Cup
Saltines	4.4	26	0.6	0.6	2 Crackers
Soy Milk	4.3	79	6.6	4.6	8oz
Club Cracker	4.2	34	0.5	1.4	2 Crackers
Ketchup	4.1	16	0.0	0.0	1 T
Ricotta, Whole	3.8	216	14.0	16.1	½ Cup
Cottage Cheese, 1%	3.1	82	14.0	1.1	4oz
Cottage Cheese	3.0	117	14.1	5.1	4oz
Garlic	3.0	13	0.6	0.0	3 Cloves
Teriyaki Sauce	2.9	15	1.1	0.0	1 T
Broccoli	2.3	12	1.3	0.0	½ Cup
Horseradish Sauce	2.3	54	0.0	4.9	1 T
Red Cabbage	2.1	10	0.5	0.0	½ Cup
Barbeque Sauce	2.0	12	0.0	0.3	1 T
Green Cabbage	1.9	8	0.4	0.0	½ Cup
Cream Cheese, Light	1.8	62	2.9	4.7	1oz
Mushrooms	1.6	9	0.7	0.0	½ Cup
Radish	1.6	7	0.3	0.0	10 Radishes
Feta Cheese	1.2	75	4.0	6.0	1oz
Swiss Cheese	1.0	107	8.1	7.8	1oz
Cheddar Cheese, Extra Sharp	1.0	100	6.0	9.0	1oz

FOOD	PROTEIN	CALORIES	CARBOHYDRATE	FAT	SERVING SIZE
PROTEIN CONTENT:					
Sorted by category					
Cereals, Cooked or to be Cooked					
Couscous	6.8	201	41.6	0.0	1Cup
Bran Rasin, Quaker	5.2	153	29.2	1.7	¾ Cooked
Oatmeal, Quick	4.4	99	18.6	2.0	⅔ Cooked
Cream of Rice	4.1	143	29.7	0.5	1 Cup
Raisins, Dates & Walnuts	4.0	141	25.1	3.8	1.3oz Dry
Total	4.0	110	22.0	2.0	1.2oz Dry
Barley, Pearled	3.6	193	44.3	0.7	1 Cup
Malt-O-Meal	3.6	100	21.1	0.4	1 Cup
Cereals, Ready to Eat					
100% Natural	13.2	508	72.0	22.0	1 Cup
Grape-Nuts	12.4	420	92.4	0.4	1 Cup
All-Bran	12.0	210	66.0	3.0	1 Cup
Corn Flakes	7.8	220	58.2	12.3	1 Cup
Oat Bran	6.2	125	25.0	2.5	1 Cup
Clusters	6.0	220	40.0	6.0	1 Cup
Fruit & Fibre	5.6	182	43.4	2.0	1 Cup
Fiber One	4.0	120	46.0	2.0	1 Cup
Bran Chex	3.8	120	30.6	0.9	1 Cup
Cheerios	3.4	88	15.6	1.4	1 Cup
Corn Bran	2.9	145	31.0	1.2	1 Cup
Apple Raisin	2.6	173	42.6	0.0	1 Cup
Rice Krispies	1.9	110	24.8	0.0	1 Cup
Cheese & Cheese Products					
Ricotta Skim	14.1	171	6.4	9.8	½ Cup
Cottage Cheese	14.1	117	3.0	5.1	4oz
Ricotta Whole	14.0	216	3.8	16.1	½ Cup
Cottage Cheese, 1%	14.0	82	3.1	1.1	4oz
Parmesan, Hard	10.1	111	0.9	7.3	1oz
Swiss	8.1	107	1.0	7.8	1oz
Provolone	7.3	100	0.6	7.6	1oz
Gouda	7.1	101	0.6	7.8	1oz
Mozzarella, Skim	6.9	72	0.8	4.5	1oz
American, Processed	6.3	106	0.5	8.9	1oz
Cheddar, Extra Sharp	6.0	100	1.0	9.0	1oz

continued

FOOD	PROTEIN	CALORIES	CARBOHYDRATE	FAT	SERVING SIZE
Mozzarella	5.5	80	0.6	6.1	1oz
Feta	4.0	75	1.2	6.0	1oz
Cream Cheese Light	2.9	62	1.8	4.7	1oz
Cream Cheese	2.3	98	0.7	9.5	1oz
Chips, Pretzels, Popcorn & Similar Snack Foods					
Trail Mix	3.9	131	12.7	8.3	1oz
Chex Mix	3.1	121	18.5	4.9	1oz
Air-Popped Popcorn	2.9	93	18.9	1.0	3 Cups
Keebler Pretzels	2.8	104	21.0	0.8	1oz
Pretzels	2.6	108	22.5	1.0	1oz
Barbecue Chips	2.2	139	15.0	9.2	1oz
Tortilla Chips	2	142	17.8	7.4	1oz
French Onion	2	170	13.0	11	1oz
Microwave Popcorn with Butter	2	90	10.0	6.0	3 Cups
Potato Sticks	1.9	148	15.1	9.8	1oz
Trail Mix Tropical	1.8	115	18.6	4.9	1oz
Eggs, Egg Dishes & Egg Substitutes					
Egg Scrambled (w/milk)	6.8	101	1.3	7.5	1 Large Egg
Boiled, Hard/Soft	6.3	77	0.6	5.3	1 Large Egg
Egg, Fried	6.2	91	0.6	6.9	1 Large Egg
Egg, Poached	6.2	74	0.6	5.0	1 Large Egg
Egg, White	3.5	17	0.0	0.0	1 Large Egg
Yolk	2.8	59	0.0	5.1	1 Large Egg
Fast Foods					
Cheeseburger, Large	30.1	608	47.4	33.0	1 Sandwich
Burrito with Beef	26.6	523	58.5	20.8	2 Burritos
Bacon Cheeseburger	25.1	464	29.1	27.3	1 Sandwich
Chicken Fillet	24.1	515	38.7	29.5	1 Sandwich
Biscuit with Egg & Ham	20.4	442	30.3	27.0	1 Biscuit
Chicken, Breaded, Fried	16.9	290	15.5	17.7	6 Pieces
Fried Chicken with Honey	16.8	329	26.9	17.5	6 Pieces
Cheeseburger, Regular	16.0	295	26.5	14.1	1 Sandwich
Burrito with Bean & Cheese	15.1	337	55.0	11.7	2 Burritos
Baked Potato with Cheese	14.6	475	46.5	28.7	1 Potato
Croissant with Egg &Cheese	12.8	369	24.3	24.7	1 Croissant
Crab Cake	11.3	160	5.1	10.4	2.1oz Cake

FOOD	PROTEIN	CALORIES	CARBOHYDRATE	FAT	SERVING SIZE
Biscuit with Egg	11.1	315	24.2	20.2	1 Biscuit
Vanilla Shake	9.8	314	50.8	8.4	10oz
Chocolate Shake	9.6	360	57.9	10.5	10oz
French Toast Sticks	8.3	479	49.1	29.1	5 Sticks
Danish Pastry, Cheese	5.8	353	28.7	24.6	3.2oz Pastry
English Muffin with Butter	4.9	189	30.3	5.8	1 Muffin
French Fries	4.6	355	44.4	18.5	Large Order
Corn on the Cob with Butter	4.5	155	32	3.4	1 Ear
Onion Rings	3.7	275	31.3	15.5	8-9 Rings
French Fries	3.0	235	29.3	12.2	Reg Order
Fish, Shellfish & Crustacea					
Tuna, White, Drained	22.7	116	0.0	2.1	3oz
Tuna, Can, Light	21.7	99	0.0	0.7	3oz
Barracuda, Raw	18.0	97	0.0	2.2	3oz
Shark, Raw	17.8	111	0.0	3.8	3oz
Halibut, Raw	17.7	93	0.0	2.0	3oz
Shrimp, Raw	17.3	90	0.8	1.5	3oz
Salmon, Raw	17.0	99	0.0	2.9	3oz
Abalone, Fried	16.7	161	9.4	5.8	3oz
Black Bass, Raw	16.4	80	0.0	1.0	3oz
Whitefish, Raw	16.2	114	0.0	5.0	3oz
Lobster, Raw	16.0	77	0.4	0.8	3oz
Sea Bass, Raw	15.7	82	0.0	1.7	3oz
Crab, Raw	15.6	71	0.0	0.5	3oz
Catfish, Raw	15.5	99	0.0	3.6	3oz
Cod, Raw	15.1	70	0.0	0.6	3oz
Abalone, Raw	14.5	89	5.1	0.6	3oz
Herring, Raw	13.9	166	0.0	11.8	3oz
Scallops, Raw	13.6	76	2.4	0.9	3oz
Octopus, Raw	12.7	70	1.9	0.9	3oz
Halibut, Breaded	11.2	165	11.2	7.5	3oz
Clams, Raw	10.9	63	2.2	0.8	3oz
Mussels, Raw	10.1	73	3.1	1.9	3oz
Lobster Salad	8.6	95	1.9	5.4	3oz
Fruit & Vegetable Juices					
Carrot Juice/bottled	2.2	97	22.8	0.4	8oz
Tomato Juice	1.8	43	10.9	0.0	8oz

continued

FOOD	PROTEIN	CALORIES	CARBOHYDRATE	FAT	SERVING SIZE
Orange Juice	1.5	104	24.5	0.4	8oz
Grapefruit Juice	1.2	96	22.7	0.0	8oz
Breads, Yeast					
Bagel	6.0	163	30.9	1.4	1 Bagel
Pita Bread/Pocket	4.0	106	20.6	0.6	1 Pocket
Honey & Oat Bran	3.2	71	12.7	1.2	1 Slice
Pumpernickel	2.9	82	15.4	0.8	1 Slice
Oatmeal	2.4	71	13.0	1.2	1 Slice
Whole Wheat	2.4	61	11.4	1.1	1 Slice
Stone Ground	2.4	48	9.9	0.7	1 Slice
Cracked Wheat	2.3	66	12.5	0.9	1 Slice
Wheat	2.3	61	11.3	1.0	1 Slice
Raisin	2.1	70	13.2	1.0	1 Slice
Rye	2.1	66	12.0	0.9	1 Slice
White	2.0	64	11.7	0.9	1 Slice
Crackers					
Breadflats	1.3	53	10.6	0.8	1 Slice
Triscuits	1.0	60	10.0	2.0	3 Crackers
Cheese Nips	1.0	70	9.0	3.0	13 Crackers
Ritz	1.0	70	9.0	4.0	4 Crackers
Wheat Thins	1.0	70	9.0	3.0	8 Crackers
Chicken in a Biskit	1.0	80	8.0	5.0	7 Crackers
Crispbread	1.0	25	5.0	0.0	1 Piece
Muffins					
English Muffin	4.5	135	26.2	1.1	1 Muffin
Bran	3.0	112	16.7	5.1	1 Muffin
Corn	2.8	130	20.0	4.2	1 Muffin
Raisin Bran	2.7	121	16.8	4.8	1 Muffin
Pasta					
Fettuccine, Spinach	17.0	360	65.0	5.0	4.5oz
Macaroni, Wheat	7.5	174	37.2	0.8	1 Cup
Macaroni, Enriched	6.7	197	39.7	0.9	1 Cup
Japanese Soba	5.8	113	24.4	0.0	1 Cup
Egg Noodles	4.5	166	30.5	1.0	4.5oz
Chow Mein	3.8	237	25.9	13.8	1 Cup

FOOD	PROTEIN	CALORIES	CARBOHYDRATE	FAT	SERVING SIZE
Meats					
Top Sirloin	29.2	229	0.0	11.6	3.5oz
Prime Rib	28.7	213	0.0	10.1	3.5oz
Veal Leg, Roasted	27.7	160	0.0	4.7	3.5oz
Extra Lean Ground	24.5	250	0.0	16.1	3.5oz
Regular Ground, Baked	23.0	287	0.0	20.9	3.5oz
Short Ribs	21.6	471	0.0	42.0	3.5oz
Ham, Roasted	20.9	145	1.5	5.5	3.5oz
Corned Beef	18.2	251	0.5	19.0	3.5oz
Smoked Sausage	14.4	311	2.6	26.6	3.5oz
Bacon Pan Fried	5.8	109	0.0	9.4	3 Med Slices
Milk, Yogurt, Milk Beverages & Milk Beverage Mixes					
Yogurt, Skim	13.0	127	17.4	0.4	8oz
Vanilla Yogurt	10.6	200	37.2	0.0	8oz
Yogurt, Skim with Fruit	10.1	200	38.2	0.0	8oz
Goat	8.7	168	10.9	10.1	8oz
Skim	8.4	86	11.9	0.4	8oz
Buttermilk Cultured	8.1	99	11.7	2.2	8oz
Low fat, 1%	8.0	102	11.7	2.6	8oz
Soy	6.6	79	4.3	4.6	8oz
Poultry					
Light Chicken w/o Skin, Roasted	30.9	173	0.0	4.5	3.5oz
Roasted Breast w/o Skin	30.9	173	0.0	4.5	3.5oz
Light Turkey w/o Skin, Roasted	29.3	170	0.0	5.0	3.5oz
Light Chicken w/o Skin, Stewed	28.9	159	0.0	4.0	3.5oz
Dark Turkey w/o Skin, Roasted	28.6	187	0.0	7.2	3.5oz
Dark Chicken w/o Skin, Roasted	27.4	205	0.0	9.7	3.5oz
Turkey, Ground	26.8	251	0.0	15.2	3.5oz
Dark Chicken w/o Skin, Stewed	26.0	192	0.0	9.0	3.5oz
Soups					
Black Bean	10.6	206	34.0	3.0	1 Cup
Green Pea	8.6	164	26.5	2.9	1 Cup
Cream of Chicken	8.3	283	22.5	17.9	1 Can
Black Bean	5.6	116	19.8	1.5	1 Cup
Beef Broth	5.5	130	24.7	1.0	1 Cup
Tomato	5.0	208	40.3	4.7	1 Can

continued

FOOD	PROTEIN	CALORIES	CARBOHYDRATE	FAT	SERVING SIZE
Cream of Mushroom	4.9	313	22.6	23.1	1 Can
Chicken Broth	4.9	39	0.9	1.4	1 Cup
Minestrone	4.3	83	11.2	2.5	1 Cup
Chicken Noodle	4.0	75	9.4	2.5	1 Cup
Turkey Noodle	3.9	69	8.6	2.0	1 Cup
Onion	3.8	57	8.2	1.7	1 Cup
Chicken Vegetable	3.6	74	8.6	2.8	1 Cup
Clam Chowder	2.2	77	12.2	2.2	1 Cup
Cream of Asparagus	2.1	81	10.4	3.5	1 Cup
Vegetables, Vegetable Products & Vegetable Salads					
Tofu	19.9	183	5.4	11.0	½ Cup
Refried Beans	7.9	135	23.4	1.3	½ Cup
Kidney Beans	7.7	112	20.2	0.4	½ Cup
Lima Beans	7.3	108	19.7	0.0	½ Cup
Baked Beans	7.0	191	27.5	6.5	½ Cup
Hummus	6.5	210	24.8	10.4	½ Cup
Artichoke	4.2	60	13.4	0.0	1 Medium
Yellow Corn	2.7	89	20.6	1.1	½ Cup
White Corn	2.4	100	21.5	0.4	½ Cup
Brussels Sprouts	2.0	30	6.8	0.4	½ Cup
Artichoke Heart	1.9	37	8.7	0.0	½ Cup
Broccoli	1.3	12	2.3	0.0	½ Cup
Green Beans	1.2	22	4.9	0.0	½ Cup
Tomato	1.0	26	5.7	0.4	1 Tomato
PROTEIN CONTENT:					
Sorted by amount					
Light Chicken w/o Skin, Roasted	30.9	173	0.0	4.5	3.5oz
Roasted Breast w/o Skin	30.9	173	0.0	4.5	3.5oz
Cheeseburger, Large	30.1	608	47.4	33.0	1 Sandwich
Light Turkey w/o Skin, Roasted	29.3	170	0.0	5.0	3.5oz
Top Sirloin	29.2	229	0.0	11.6	3.5oz
Light Chicken w/o Skin, Stewed	28.9	159	0.0	4.0	3.5oz
Prime Rib	28.7	213	0.0	10.1	3.5oz
Dark Turkey w/o Skin, Roasted	28.6	187	0.0	7.2	3.5oz
Veal Leg, Roasted	27.7	160	0.0	4.7	3.5oz
Dark Chicken w/o Skin, Roasted	27.4	205	0.0	9.7	3.5oz
Turkey, Ground	26.8	251	0.0	15.2	3.5oz

FOOD	PROTEIN	CALORIES	CARBOHYDRATE	FAT	SERVING SIZE
Burrito with Beef	26.6	523	58.5	20.8	2 Burritos
Dark Chicken w/o Skin, Stewed	26.0	192	0.0	9.0	3.5oz
Bacon Cheeseburger	25.1	464	29.1	27.3	1 Sandwich
Extra Lean Ground	24.5	250	0.0	16.1	3.5oz
Chicken Fillet	24.1	515	38.7	29.5	1 Sandwich
Regular Ground, Baked	23.0	287	0.0	20.9	3.5oz
Tuna, White, Drained	22.7	116	0.0	2.1	3oz
Tuna, Can, Light	21.7	99	0.0	0.7	3oz
Short Ribs	21.6	471	0.0	42.0	3.5oz
Ham, Roasted	20.9	145	1.5	5.5	3.5oz
Biscuit with Egg & Ham	20.4	442	30.3	27.0	1 Biscuit
Tofu	19.9	183	5.4	11.0	½ Cup
Corned Beef	18.2	251	0.5	19.0	3.5oz
Barracuda, Raw	18.0	97	0.0	2.2	3oz
Shark, Raw	17.8	111	0.0	3.8	3oz
Halibut, Raw	17.7	93	0.0	2.0	3oz
Shrimp, Raw	17.3	90	0.8	1.5	3oz
Salmon, Raw	17.0	99	0.0	2.9	3oz
Fettuccine, Spinach	17.0	360	65.0	5.0	4.5oz
Chicken, Breaded, Fried	16.9	290	15.5	17.7	6 Pieces
Fried Chicken with Honey	16.8	329	26.9	17.5	6 Pieces
Abalone, Fried	16.7	161	9.4	5.8	3oz
Black Bass, Raw	16.4	79.7	0.0	1.0	3oz
Whitefish, Raw	16.2	114	0.0	5.0	3oz
Cheeseburger, Regular	16.0	295	26.5	14.1	1 Sandwich
Lobster, Raw	16.0	77	0.4	0.8	3oz
Sea Bass, Raw	15.7	82	0.0	1.7	3oz
Crab, Raw	15.6	71	0.0	0.5	3oz
Catfish, Raw	15.5	99	0.0	3.6	3oz
Burrito with Bean & Cheese	15.1	337	55.0	11.7	2 Burritos
Cod, Raw	15.1	70	0.0	0.6	3oz
Baked Potato with Cheese	14.6	475	46.5	28.7	1 Potato
Abalone, Raw	14.5	89	5.1	0.6	3oz
Smoked Sausage	14.4	311	2.6	26.6	3.5oz
Cottage Cheese	14.1	117	3.0	5.1	4oz
Ricotta Skim	14.1	171	6.4	9.8	½ Cup
Cottage Cheese, 1%	14.0	82	3.1	1.1	4oz
Ricotta, Whole	14.0	216	3.8	16.1	½ Cup

continued

FOOD	PROTEIN	CALORIES	CARBOHYDRATE	FAT	SERVING SIZE
Herring, Raw	13.9	166	0.0	11.8	3oz
Scallops, Raw	13.6	75.4	2.4	0.9	3oz
100% Natural Granola	13.2	508	72.0	22.0	1 Cup
Yogurt, Skim	13.0	127	17.4	0.4	8oz
Croissant with Egg & Cheese	12.8	369	24.3	24.7	1 Croissant
Octopus, Raw	12.7	70	1.9	0.9	3oz
Grape-Nuts	12.4	420	92.4	0.4	1 Cup
All-Bran	12.0	210	66.0	3.0	1 Cup
Crab Cake	11.3	160	5.1	10.4	2.1oz Cake
Halibut, Breaded	11.2	165	11.2	7.5	3oz
Biscuit with Egg	11.1	315	24.2	20.2	1 Biscuit
Clams, Raw	10.9	63	2.2	0.8	3oz
Vanilla Yogurt	10.6	200	37.2	0.0	8oz
Black Bean Soup	10.6	206	34.0	3.0	1 Cup
Parmesan, Hard	10.1	111	0.9	7.3	1oz
Mussels, Raw	10.1	73	3.1	1.9	3oz
Yogurt, Skim with Fruit	10.1	200	38.2	0.0	8oz
Vanilla Shake	9.8	314	50.8	8.4	10oz
Chocolate Shake	9.6	360	57.9	10.5	10oz
Goat Milk	8.7	168	10.9	10.1	8oz
Lobster Salad	8.6	94	1.9	5.4	3oz
Green Pea Soup	8.6	164	26.5	2.9	1 Cup
Skim Milk	8.4	86	11.9	0.4	8oz
French Toast Sticks	8.3	479	49.1	29.1	5 Sticks
Cream of Chicken	8.3	283	22.5	17.9	1 Can
Swiss Cheese	8.1	107	1.0	7.8	1oz
Buttermilk, Cultured	8.1	99	11.7	2.2	8oz
Low-fat Milk, 1%	8.0	102	11.7	2.6	8oz
Refried Beans	7.9	135	23.4	1.3	½ Cup
Corn Flakes	7.8	220	58.2	12.3	1 Cup
Kidney Beans	7.7	112	20.2	0.4	½ Cup
Macaroni, Wheat	7.5	174	37.2	0.8	1 Cup
Provolone	7.3	100	0.6	7.6	1oz
Lima Beans	7.3	108	19.7	0.3	½ Cup
Gouda	7.1	101	0.6	7.8	1oz
Baked Beans	7.0	191	27.5	6.5	½ Cup
Mozzarella, Skim	6.9	72	0.8	4.5	1oz
Couscous	6.8	201	41.6	0.0	1 Cup

FOOD	PROTEIN	CALORIES	CARBOHYDRATE	FAT	SERVING SIZE
Egg Scrambled (w/Milk)	6.8	101	1.3	7.5	1 Large Egg
Macaroni, Enriched	6.7	197	39.7	0.9	1 Cup
Soy Milk	6.6	79	4.3	4.6	8oz
Hummus	6.5	210	24.8	10.4	½ Cup
American, Processed	6.3	106	0.5	8.9	1oz
Boiled, Hard/Soft	6.3	77	0.6	5.3	1 Large Egg
Oat Bran	6.2	125	25.0	2.5	1 Cup
Egg, Fried	6.2	91	0.6	6.9	1 Large Egg
Egg, Poached	6.2	74	0.6	5.0	1 Large Egg
Clusters Cereal	6.0	220	40.0	6.0	1 Cup
Cheddar Cheese, Extra Sharp	6.0	100	1.0	9.0	1oz
Bagel	6.0	163	30.9	1.4	1 Bagel
Danish Pastry Cheese	5.8	353	28.7	24.6	3.2oz Pastry
Japanese Soba	5.8	113	24.4	0.0	1 Cup
Bacon, Pan Fried	5.8	109	0.0	9.4	3 Med Slices
Fruit & Fibre Cereal	5.6	182	43.4	2.0	1 Cup
Black Bean Soup	5.6	116	19.8	1.5	1 Cup
Mozzarella Cheese	5.5	80	0.6	6.1	1oz
Beef Broth	5.5	130	24.7	1.0	1 Cup
Bran Raisin, Quaker	5.2	153	29.2	1.7	¾ Cooked
Tomato Soup	5.0	208	40.3	4.7	1 Can
English Muffin with Butter	4.9	189	30.3	5.8	1 Muffin
Cream of Mushroom	4.9	313	22.6	23.1	1 Can
Chicken Broth	4.9	39	0.9	1.4	1 Cup
French Fries	4.6	355	44.4	18.5	Large Order
Corn on the Cob with Butter	4.5	155	32.0	3.4	1 Ear
English Muffin	4.5	135	26.2	1.1	1 Muffin
Egg Noodles	4.5	166	30.5	1.0	4.5oz
Oatmeal, Quick	4.4	99	18.6	2.0	⅔ Cooked
Minestrone	4.3	83	11.2	2.5	1 Cup
Artichoke	4.2	60	13.4	0.0	1 Medium
Cream of Rice Soup	4.1	143	29.7	0.5	1Cup
Raisins, Dates & Walnuts	4.0	141	25.1	3.8	1.3oz Dry
Total	4.0	110	22.0	2.0	1.2oz Dry
Fiber One	4.0	120	46.0	2.0	1 Cup
Feta Cheese	4.0	75	1.2	6.0	1oz
Pita Bread/Pocket	4.0	106	20.6	0.6	1 Pocket
Chicken Noodle Soup	4.0	75	9.4	2.5	1 Cup

continued

FOOD	PROTEIN	CALORIES	CARBOHYDRATE	FAT	SERVING SIZE
Trail Mix	3.9	131	12.7	8.3	1oz
Turkey Noodle Soup	3.9	69	8.6	2.0	1 Cup
Bran Chex	3.8	120	30.6	0.9	1 Cup
Chow Mein	3.8	237	25.9	13.8	1 Cup
Onion Soup	3.8	57	8.2	1.7	1 Cup
Onion Rings	3.7	275	31.3	15.5	8-9 Rings
Barley, Pearled	3.6	193	44.3	0.7	1Cup
Malt-O-Meal	3.6	100	21.1	0.4	1Cup
Chicken Vegetable Soup	3.6	74	8.6	2.8	1 Cup
Egg White	3.5	17	0.0	0.0	1 Large Egg
Cheerios	3.4	88	15.6	1.4	1 Cups
Honey & Oat Bran	3.2	71	12.7	1.2	1 Slice
Chex Mix	3.1	121	18.5	4.9	1oz
French Fries	3.0	235	29.3	12.2	Reg Order
Bran	3.0	112	16.7	5.1	1 Muffin
Corn Bran	2.9	145	31.0	1.2	1 Cup
Cream Cheese, Light	2.9	62	1.8	4.7	1oz
Air-Popped Popcorn	2.9	92.5	18.9	1.0	3 Cups
Pumpernickel	2.9	82	15.4	0.8	1 Slice
Keebler Pretzels	2.8	104	21.0	0.8	1oz
Yolk	2.8	59	0.0	5.1	1 Large Egg
Corn Muffin	2.8	130	20	4.2	1 Muffin
Raisin Bran Muffin	2.7	121	16.8	4.8	1 Muffin
Yellow Corn	2.7	89	20.6	1.1	½ Cup
Apple Raisin	2.6	173	42.6	0	1 Cup
Pretzels	2.6	108	22.5	1.0	1oz
Oatmeal Bread	2.4	71	13	1.2	1 Slice
Whole Wheat Bread	2.4	61	11.4	1.1	1 Slice
Stone Ground Bread	2.4	48	9.9	0.7	1 Slice
White Corn	2.4	100	21.5	0.4	½ Cup
Cream Cheese	2.3	98	0.7	9.5	1oz
Cracked Wheat	2.3	66	12.5	0.9	1 Slice
Wheat	2.3	61	11.3	1.0	1 Slice
Barbecue Chips	2.2	139	15	9.2	1oz
Carrot Juice	2.2	97	22.8	0.4	8oz
Clam Chowder	2.2	77	12.2	2.2	1 Cup
Raisin Bread	2.1	70	13.2	1.0	1 Slice
Rye Bread	2.1	66	12.0	0.9	1 Slice

FOOD	PROTEIN	CALORIES	CARBOHYDRATE	FAT	SERVING SIZE
Cream of Asparagus Soup	2.1	81	10.4	3.5	1 Cup
French Onion Chips	2.0	170	13.0	11.0	1oz
Tortilla Chips	2.0	142	17.8	7.4	1oz
Microwave Popcorn with Butter	2.0	90	10.0	6.0	3 Cups
White Bread	2.0	64	11.7	0.9	1 Slice
Brussels Sprouts	2.0	30	6.8	0.4	½ Cup
Rice Krispies	1.9	110	24.8	0.0	1 Cup
Potato Sticks	1.9	148	15.1	9.8	1oz
Papaya, Raw	1.9	117	29.8	0.4	1 Medium
Artichoke Heart	1.9	37	8.7	0.0	½ Cup
Trail Mix Tropical	1.8	115	18.6	4.9	1oz
Tomato Juice	1.8	43	10.9	0.0	8oz
Dates, Dried	1.6	228	61.0	0.4	10 Dates
Orange Juice	1.5	104	24.5	0.4	8oz
Orange	1.4	65	16.3	0.0	1 Medium
Cantaloupe, Raw	1.4	57	13.4	0.4	1 Cup
Grapefruit/Bottled	1.3	93	22.1	0.0	8oz
Breadflats	1.3	53	10.6	0.8	1 Slice
Broccoli	1.3	12	2.3	0.0	½ Cup
Grapefruit Juice	1.2	96	22.7	0.0	8oz
Green Beans	1.2	22	4.9	0.0	½ Cup
Cheese Nips	1.0	70	9.0	3.0	13 Crackers
Chicken in a Biskit	1.0	80	8.0	5.0	7 Crackers
Ritz	1.0	70	9.0	4.0	4 Crackers
Triscuits	1.0	60	10.0	2.0	3 Crackers
Wheat Thins	1.0	70	9.0	3.0	8 Crackers
Crispbread	1.0	25	5.0	0.0	1 Piece
Tomato	1.0	26	5.7	0.4	1 Tomato

High Octane Fuel

Think of your body for a moment as if it were a car. Before you can drive it, you have to make sure there's gas in the engine. When you turn the car on, you start burning the gas. The energy that results powers the car.

Your body is not all that different. Before it can perform even the slightest movement or task, it needs energy. That energy ultimately comes from the carbohydrates and fats (fatty acids) that you eat. Blood glucose derived from dietary carbohydrates is the primary fuel used by the cells of our body.

The process of energy conversion from food is one of the most technical processes described in this book. When you understand the process, you'll have a better understanding of how to pace yourself in a workout.

How the Body Converts the Food You Eat into Energy

In order to convert essential nutrients into energy, your body has to first break the food down into a high-energy molecule called adenosine triphosphate, or ATP. As ATP is broken down, it releases chemical energy used to perform bodily work—muscle contractions, movement, or any form of work necessary for survival. In addition to producing energy, the process also produces heat, which is why your body temperature goes up when you exercise.

Like the gas burning in a car, the conversion of food in your body produces by-products, one of which is called adenosine diphosphate (ADP). ADP is later reformed back into ATP from other energy stores in the body, including glucose and free fatty acids.

As with the gasoline in your gas tank, your body can only store limited amounts of ATP (enough for only several seconds of exercise). Because it has such a limited supply, the body has to continually resynthesize and resupply ATP to the muscles if movement or repair is to continue. The process your body uses to release energy is called catabolism. Catabolism has three different processes. The first supplies energy immediately at the onset of exercise. The second supplies energy during short-term, high-intensity exercise; and the third delivers energy over longer periods of time.

The first two are anaerobic, because they don't require oxygen. Immediate energy release, called the phosphagen or ATP-CP system, uses the small amounts of ATP and another high-energy compound called creatine phosphate (CP) that is stored in limited amounts in the muscles. Because the muscles can only store minute quantities of ATP and because creatine phosphate can only resynthesize ATP for 10 seconds, you can only draw on this energy for those

10 seconds. As a result, the ATP-CP system is perfect for that sudden burst of sudden energy you need on a go-for-broke sprint, for climbing hills, swinging a golf club or tennis racquet, or lifting a weight.

As this small quantity of stored ATP and CP are exhausted, the body shifts into its second mode of energy production, the burning of short-term anaerobic fuel. This second system, which is called glycolysis, breaks down glucose or glycogen in the muscle. As it does, it releases the energy necessary to resynthesize ATP and CP from ADP and creatine, respectively.

The process also releases a by-product called lactic acid. Because glycolysis is an anaerobic system and thus operates without oxygen, the lactic acid cannot be efficiently oxidized, and builds up in the muscles. As it accumulates, the lactic acid begins leaking into the bloodstream. Within several minutes, there is enough excess lactic acid in the blood to cause a burning pain in the muscle. Soon thereafter, the lactic acid levels are high enough to prevent your muscle from contracting for more than a few seconds.

These two systems can only provide short bursts of energy because they draw upon limited stores of ATP or anaerobically metabolized glucose, which leads to the buildup of lactic acid, forcing the muscles to stop exercising. To obtain energy for longer workouts or activities, the body depends upon the third system, the aerobic system.

Aerobic metabolism relies on carbohydrates and fats (and to a minor degree, protein). Generally, it burns the carbohydrates and fats in an inverse relationship: The higher the intensity of the exercise, the more the body relies on carbohydrates, rather than fat. Similarly, the more moderate the exercise, the more the body relies on fat sources, rather than carbohydrates for energy.

Low- or High-Intensity Exercise to Burn Fat & Calories?

Given a comparable amount of time to spend exercising and the following information, you can see it is better to train at a higher intensity (within one's target heart rate zone) to utilize both fat and total calories. This example compares both the fat and the total calories expended during 30 minutes of continuous exercise at either 50 percent or 70 percent of one's maximal aerobic capacity (VO_2max). The individual's VO_2max for this example is measured at 3.0 liters O_2 / minute. The following is the percent contribution of calories from fat or carbohydrate for energy production at selected exercise intensities:

INTENSITY	% CALORIES FROM FAT	% CALORIES FROM CARBOHYDRATE
rest	60	40
50% VO_2max	50	50
70% VO_2max	40	60

Example:

EXERCISE INTENSITY	CALORIES EXPENDED	
	TOTAL	FAT
@ 50% VO_2max	225 calories (50% x 3.0 x 5* x 30)	112.5 calories (50% x 225)
@ 70% VO_2max	315 calories (70% x 3.0 x 5* x 30)	126 calories (40% x 225)

*By measuring the amount of oxygen the body consumes, it is possible to determine the calories of energy being expended during different activities. For every liter of oxygen consumed, five calories of energy are expended.

Conclusion: A higher exercise intensity not only utilizes more total calories, but also more fat calories. While fewer (relative) fat calories are utilized at a higher exercise intensity, more total fat calories are utilized as long as the total exercise duration is similar and within the training sensitive (aerobic) exercise zone.

That has led to some confusion in the media, and has steered some people, particularly those interested in weight loss, away from high-intensity exercise. But that is a mistake, if only because exercise is not an either/or situation. The calories you burn during a workout are taken from both carbohydrates and fat. At high intensities, you burn a greater percentage of carbohydrates than fat; at lower levels, you burn a greater percentage of fat. But because higher-intensity exercise burns substantially more calories than low- or moderate-intensity exercise, you burn more actual fat calories.

The aerobic system can deliver energy over a prolonged duration, but it cannot be switched on immediately. It takes several minutes of exercise, as well as an increased respiration and heart rate, to deliver enough oxygen to the working muscle cells for aerobic catabolism to begin. That is why a warm-up is so important—it gives the body a chance to prepare for and ease into the aerobic state.

A BREAKDOWN OF THE ENERGY SYSTEMS

SYSTEM	DURATION	FUEL	TYPICAL SPORT
ATP-CP, ANAEROBIC	UP TO 10 SECONDS	ATP, CP	WEIGHT LIFTING, TENNIS SERVE, GOLF SWING
SHORT TERM, ANAEROBIC	SEVERAL MINUTES	GLUCOSE, GLYCOGEN	SPRINTS, WEIGHT TRAINING HILL CLIMBS
LONG TERM, AEROBIC	UP TO SEVERAL HOURS	GLUCOSE, GLYCOGEN, FATTY ACIDS, TRIGLYCERIDES	AEROBIC DANCE, ENDURANCE RUNS OR RIDES, CROSS-COUNTRY SKIING, TENNIS MATCH

As with the burning of carbohydrates and fat, we can talk about these three systems as if they were independent. In reality, however, they operate in tandem. Until the aerobic system is switched on, the burden of energy supply falls on the anaerobic energy systems. As the aerobic system kicks in, the other two function at lower levels. In the aerobic system, the muscles still produce lactic acid, although there is enough oxygen and ATP in the muscles and liver to oxidize and metabolize it so muscles are able to continue to function. If you have to surpass the capacity of the aerobic system, such as when you have to ride your bike up a steep hill or run away from a snarling dog, you immediately switch into available ATP and CP and seconds later into short-term energy sources.

Remember that both anaerobic pathways of energy production can only supply energy for short amounts of time. If you don't cut back, lactic acid buildup will force you to stop. To maintain the activity, you have to ease into a moderate pace, which allows the long-term, aerobic energy system to predominate.

Since you are the best judge of your position in the energy spectrum, you can use this information to pace yourself during aerobic activities. If you're reaching your aerobic limit, decrease the intensity so you can continue the workout or complete the event. If you are almost done, you can continue at the same pace for a short time, then your body will force you to stop.

Resources

Numerous resources exist for finding reliable nutrition information. Below you will find a partial list of some credible agencies, groups, organizations, books, journals, and websites on nutrition.

Agencies/Groups/Organizations:

American College of Sports Medicine
PO Box 1440
Indianapolis, IN 46206–1440
(317) 637–9200

American Dietetic Association
216 West Jackson Boulevard, Suite 800
Chicago, IL 60606-6995
(312) 899-0040

Center for Science in the Public Interest
1875 Connecticut Avenue, NW, Suite 300
Washington, DC 20009
(202) 332-9110

Food and Drug Administration
Office of Consumer Affairs
5600 Fishers Lane
Rockville, MD 20857
(301) 443-3170

Food and Nutrition Information Center
10301 Baltimore Boulevard, Room 304
Beltsville, MD 20705
(301) 504-5719

National Council Against Health Fraud, Inc.
PO Box 1276
Loma Linda, CA 92354-9983
(714) 824-4690

Books:

Exercise Physiology: Energy, Nutrition, and Human Performance, 4th edition, William D. McArdle, Frank I. Katch and Victor L. Katch, Williams & Wilkins, Baltimore, MD, 1996.

Nutrition for Health, Fitness & Sport, 5th Edition, Melvin H. Williams, WCB McGraw-Hill, Boston, MA, 1999.

Nutrition in Exercise and Sport, editors James F. Hickson and Ira Wolinsky, CRC Press, Boca Raton, FL, 1990.

Sports & Exercise Nutrition, William D. McArdle, Frank I. Katch and Victor L. Katch, Lippincott Williams & Wilkins, Baltimore, MD, 1999.

Scientific journals:

Acta Physiologica Scandinavica
American Journal of Clinical
  Nutrition
American Journal of Sports Medicine
European Journal of Applied
  Physiology

FDA Consumer
Human Nutrition: Applied Nutrition
International Journal of Obesity
International Journal of Sport Nutrition
Journal of the American Dietetic
  Association

Journal of the American Medical
  Association
Journal of Applied Physiology
Journal of Nutrition Education
Journal of Sports Medicine
Journal of Strength Conditioning
Medicine and Science in Sports and
  Exercise

Nutrition and Metabolism
Nutrition Today
Sports Medicine
Strength and Conditioning Journal
The Journal of Nutrition

Websites:

vm.cfsan.fda.gov/list.html
ipl.sils.umich.edu/ref/RR/
www.acsm.org
www.cspinet.org
www.fda.gov
www.nalusda.gov/fnic/

www.gssiweb.com
www.nal.usda.gov/fnic/foodcomp
www.nih.www.quackwatch.comgov/icd/
www.simplyfit.com
www.sportcare.com
www. sportsmedicine.com

Glossary

This glossary includes terms used in this book or ones that are generally used in the areas of sports nutrition, diet or exercise.

Acclimatization: adaptation to an environmental condition such as heat or altitude.

Adaptation: the adjustment of the body to its environment, or the process by which it enhances such fitness.

Adenosine Triphosphate (ATP): high-energy compound formed from oxidation of fat and carbohydrate. Used as energy supply for muscle and other body functions; the energy currency.

Adequacy: characterizes a diet that provides all of the essential nutrients, fiber, and energy (calories) in amounts sufficient to maintain health.

Adipocyte: a fat cell composed primarily of fat (triglycerides).

Adipose: fat tissue.

Adrenaline (epinephrine): hormone from the adrenal medulla and nerve endings of the sympathetic nervous system; secreted during times of stress to help mobilize energy.

Aerobic: requiring oxygen.

Aerobic Fitness: maximum ability to take in, transport, and utilize oxygen.

Aerobic Training: cardiovascular exercise, continuous vigorous exercise requiring the body to increase its consumption of oxygen and develop the muscles' ability to sustain activity over a long period of time.

Agility: ability to change direction quickly while maintaining control of the body.

Amenorrhea: failure to menstruate, reflecting a halted ovulatory cycle.

Amino Acids: building blocks of protein; each is a nitrogen containing compound with an amine group at one end, an acid group at the other, and a distinctive side chain.

Anabolism: cells making complex molecules from simpler compounds, opposite of catabolism.

Anaerobic: not requiring oxygen.

Anaerobic Threshold: more properly called onset of blood lactate accumulate (OBLA), as well as lactate threshold; the point at which lactate produced in working muscles begins to accumulate in the blood. Defines the upper limit of exercise that can be sustained aerobically.

Antioxidant: a compound that protects other compounds from oxygen by itself reacting with oxygen; a substance, such as a vitamin, that is "anti-oxygen"—it helps to prevent damage done to the body as a result of chemical reactions that involve the use of oxygen.

Appetite: the psychological desire to find and eat food, experienced as a pleasant sensation, often in absence of hunger.

Artificial Sweeteners: nonnutritive sugar replacements such as acesulfame K, aspartame, and saccharin.

Aspartame: a dipeptide containing the amino acids aspartic acid and phenylalanine. While it is digested as protein and supplies calories, it is so sweet that only small amounts, which contribute negligible calories, are needed to sweeten foods.

Atherosclerosis: a type of cardiovascular disease; the most common kind of hardening of the arteries characterized by the formation of fatty deposits, or plaques, in their inner walls.

Athlete: anyone participating in exercise, sports, or games requiring physical strength, agility, or endurance.

Atrophy: a decrease in size in response to disuse.

Balance: a feature of a diet that provides a number of types of foods in balance with one another, such that foods rich in one nutrient do not crowd out the foods that are rich in another nutrient.

Balanced meal: a meal containing sufficient but not excessive amounts of foods from each of the food groups and therefore sufficient but not excessive amounts of carbohydrate, protein, fat, vitamin, and mineral.

Basal Metabolic Rate (BMR): the rate at which the body spends energy to support its basal metabolism. The BMR accounts for the largest component of a person's daily energy (calorie) needs.

Basal Metabolism: the sum total of all the chemical activities of the cells necessary to sustain life, exclusive of voluntary activities. The ongoing activities of the cells when the body is at rest.

Behavior Modification: a process developed by psychologists for helping people make lasting behavior changes.

Bioavailability: the degree to which the body is able to use a substance in the form or amount present in the diet.

Body Composition: the component parts of the body—mainly fat and fat-free weight.

Branched-chain Amino Acid (BCAA): a group of three essential amino acids: isoleucine, leucine, and valine, used preferentially during exercise as a nitrogen source for energy catabolism.

Brown sugar: white sugar with molasses added; about 95 percent pure sucrose.

Buffer: substance in blood that soaks up hydrogen ions to minimize changes in acid-base balance.

Caffeine: a type of compound, called a methylxanthine, found in coffee beans, cola nuts, cocoa beans, and tea leaves. A central nervous system stimulant, caffeine's effects include increasing the heart rate, boosting urine production, raising blood triglycerides, and raising the metabolic rate.

Calorie: the unit used to measure energy. Technically, when we see the term "calorie" on food labels or talk about the amount of calories our bodies need or which we burn during activities, we are referring to kilocalories (kcal)—the amount of heat required to raise the temperature of one kilogram of water one degree Celsius.

Carbohydrates: compounds made of simple sugars or multiples of them composed of carbon, hydrogen, and oxygen atoms. Carbo = carbon (C), hydrate = water (H_2O). Some important carbohydrates are the starches, fibers, and sugars. Carbohydrates are one of the basic foodstuffs.

Carcinogen: cancer-causing substance.

Catabolism: breakdown of food compounds into smaller compounds generally for energy; opposite of anabolism, the other phase of metabolism.

Cholesterol: one type of fat, a sterol, manufactured in the body for a variety of purposes and also found in animal-derived foods.

Chylomicron: a type of lipoprotein (very low in density) made by the cells of the intestinal wall; serves as a means of transporting newly digested fat from the intestine through lymph and blood. Chylomicrons donate lipids (triglycerides) to all body cells, and primarily fat cells, and the remnants are ultimately cleared from the blood by liver cells.

Coenzymes: enzyme helpers; small molecules that interact with enzymes and enable them to do their work. Many coenzymes are made from water-soluble vitamins.

Cofactor: a mineral element that, like a coenzyme, works with an enzyme to facilitate a chemical reaction.

Complementary Proteins: two or more food proteins whose amino acid assortments complement each other in such a way that the essential amino acids limited or missing from each are supplied by the other.

Complete Proteins: proteins containing all the essential amino acids in the right proportion relative to need. The quality of a protein is judged by the proportions of essential amino acids that it contains relative to our needs.

Complex Carbohydrates: long chains of sugars (glucose arranged as starch or fiber. Also called polysaccharides.)

Concentrated Fruit Juice Sweetener: a concentrated sugar syrup made from dehydrated, deflavored fruit juice, used to sweeten products that can then claim to be "all fruit."

Concentric: muscle contractions that involve shortening of the contracted muscle.

Contraction: development of tension by muscle; concentric—muscle shortens; eccentric—muscle lengthens under tension; isometric (static)—contraction without change in length.

Corn Sweeteners: corn syrup and sugar derived from corn.

Cortisol: the main glucocorticoid hormone secreted by the adrenal glands in response to stress.

Creatine Phosphate (CP): energy-rich compound that backs up ATP in providing energy for muscles.

Daily values (DV): the amount of fat, sodium, fiber and other nutrients health experts say should make up a healthful diet. The percent daily values that appear on food labels tell you the percentage of a nutrient that a serving of the food contributed to a healthful diet.

Dehydration: the condition resulting from excessive loss of body water.

Delayed-Onset Muscle Soreness (DOMS): muscle soreness that peaks 24 to 48 hours after unfamiliar exercise or vigorous eccentric contractions.

Dextrose: another name for glucose.

Diabetes: a disorder characterized by insufficiency or relative ineffectiveness of insulin, which renders a person unable to regulate the blood glucose level normally.

Disaccharide: A double sugar composed of two monosaccharide units. Sucrose, or table sugar is composed of one glucose molecule and one fructose molecule bound together. Two other common disaccharides are lactose, milk sugar, composed of one galactose molecule and one glucose molecule, and maltose, made up of two glucose molecules bound together.

Disease: any significant abnormality in the body's structure or function that disrupts a person's vital function or physical, mental, or social well-being.

Eccentric: contraction that involves lengthening of a contracted muscle working against gravity or momentum.

Electrolyte: solution of ions (sodium, potassium) that conducts an electrical current.

Empty-Calorie Foods: a phrase used to indicate a food that supplies calories but negligible nutrients. When many empty-calorie foods are eaten regularly, they displace nutrient-dense foods from the diet and contribute to both poor nutritional health and obesity.

Endogenous: arising from causes on or within the body.

Endurance: the ability to sustain an effort for a long time. One type, muscle endurance, is the ability of a muscle to contract repeatedly within a given time without becoming exhausted. Another type, cardiovascular endurance, is the ability of the cardiovascular system to sustain effort over a period of time.

Endurance (Aerobic) Training: a form of conditioning designed to increase aerobic capacity and endurance performance.

Energy: the capacity or ability to perform work, measured in calories.

Energy Balance: the balance that results when caloric expenditure equals caloric intake.

Enzyme: biochemical catalyst allowing chemical reactions to take place.

Epinephrine: see Adrenaline.

Ergogenic aid: special substances or treatments used in attempts to improve physiological, psychological, or biomechanical functions important to sport; ergogenic refers to an increase in the rate of work output.

Essential Amino Acids: amino acids that cannot be synthesized by the body or that cannot be synthesized in amounts sufficient to meet physiological need.

Essential Nutrients: nutrients that must be obtained from food because the body cannot make them for itself.

Etiology: theory, or study, of the factors involved in causing a disease.

Evaporation: elimination of body heat when sweat vaporizes on surface of skin; evaporation of 1 L of sweat yields a heat loss of 580 calories.

Exogenous: originating outside of the body.

Fat Cell Theory: states that during the growing years, fat cells respond to overfeeding by producing additional cells (hyperplastic obesity); the number of fat cells eventually becomes fixed. With reduction in body weight, fat cell number remains constant while their size decreases. Overfeeding in adulthood causes the body to enlarge existing fat cells (hypertrophic obesity). Hypertrophic obesity is the more common type, and is usually seen in adults.

Fats: a foodstuff containing glycerol and three fatty acids; lipids that are solid at room temperature.

Fatty Acids: basic units of fat composed of chains of carbon atoms. They are either saturated with hydrogen atoms are unsaturated.

Fat-Free Weight: that portion of the body weight remaining when the weight of body fat is subtracted from the total body weight; mainly the weight of the skeletal muscle mass.

Fatigue: loss of muscle power or weakness. Diminished work capacity, usually short of true physiological limits. Real limits in short, intense exercise—factors within muscle (low pH, calcium, etc.); in long duration exercise—glycogen depletion or central nervous system fatigue due to low blood sugar.

Fibers: the indigestible residues of food, composed mostly of polysaccharides. Thus fibers are the nonstarch polysaccharides in foods.

Fitness: the body's ability to meet physical demands composed of four components: flexibility, strength, muscle endurance, and cardiovascular endurance.

Flexibility: the ability to bend or extend without injury; flexibility depends on the elasticity of muscles, tendons, and ligaments and on the condition of the joints.

Food Additive: any substance added to food, including substances used in the production, processing, treatment, packaging, transportation, or storage of food.

Food Composition Tables: tables that list the nutrient profile of commonly eaten foods.

Foodstuff: a substance suitable for food.

Fortified Food: a food to which manufacturers have added 10 percent or more of the Daily Value for a particular nutrient.

Free Radical: a highly toxic compound created in the body as a result of chemical reactions that involve oxygen. Environmental pollutants such as cigarette smoke and ozone also prompt the formation of free radicals.

Frequency: number of times per day or week in the case of exercise prescription.

Fructose: fruit sugar, the sweetest of the simple sugars (monosaccharides).

Glucagon: insulin's opposing hormone, released by the pancreas when blood glucose is too low; it raises blood glucose levels by stimulating the liver to break down stored carbohydrate, glycogen, into glucose and releasing it into the blood making it available to supply energy needs to cells.

Glucose: the building block of carbohydrate; a single sugar used in both plant and animal tissue as quick-energy currency.

Glycerol: an organic compound, three carbons long, of interest here because it serves as the backbone of triglycerides.

Glycogen: a polysaccharide composed of chains of glucose, manufactured in the body and stored in liver and muscle. As a storage form of glucose, glycogen can be broken down by the liver to maintain a constant blood glucose level when carbohydrate intake is inadequate.

Granulated Sugar: common table sugar; 99.9 percent pure sucrose.

Health: physical, mental, and social well-being; the absence of disease.

Heartburn: esophageal pain caused by backflow of stomach acid into esophagus.

Heart Disease: any of the group of cardiac disorders that together constitute the leading cause of death in the United States.

Heart Rate: the number of times the heart beats per minute.

Heat Stress: temperature-humidity combination that leads to heat disorders such as heat cramps, heat exhaustion, or heat stroke.

High-Density Lipoprotein (HDL): termed "good" cholesterol; carries cholesterol in the blood back to the liver for recycling or disposal.

High-Fructose Corn Syrup: the predominant sweetener used in processed foods and beverages; contains mostly fructose, with some glucose and maltose.

Homeostasis: relative uniformity of the normal body's internal environment.

Honey: primarily a mixture of glucose and fructose made by bees from the sucrose in nectar.

Hormones: chemical messengers. Hormones are secreted by a variety of glands in the body in response to altered conditions. Each affects one or more target tissues or organs and elicits specific responses to restore normal conditions.

Hunger: the physiological drive to find and eat food, experienced as an unpleasant sensation.

Hydrogenation: the process of adding hydrogen to unsaturated fat to make it more solid and more resistant to chemical change. In the process of partial hydrogenization trans-fatty acids are formed.

Hypercholesterolemia: excess cholesterol in the blood. Desirable level is below 200 mg/dl.

Hyperglycemia: an abnormally high blood glucose concentration, often a symptom of diabetes.

Hypertension: abnormally high blood pressure, usually higher than 140/90 mm Hg.

Hypertrophy: an increase in size in response to use.

Hypoglycemia: an abnormally low blood glucose concentration—below 60 to 70 mg/100 ml.

Ideal Body Weight: estimated weight considered best for optimal health and/or performance based on age, height, and body composition.

Immune System: the body's defense system against disease.

Incomplete Protein: a protein lacking or low in one or more of the essential amino acids.

Insoluble Fiber: includes the fiber types called cellulose, hemicellulose, and lignin; insoluble fibers do not dissolve in water. Found primarily in grains, wheat products, and vegetables.

Insulin: a hormone secreted by the pancreas in response to high blood glucose levels; it assists fat and muscle cell in drawing glucose from the blood.

Intensity: the relative rate, speed, or level of exertion.

Interval Training: training method that alternates short bouts of intense effort with periods of active rest.

Isoflavones: compounds found in many fruits, vegetables, and soy-based foods that are thought to play a role in fighting cancers.

Isokinetic: contraction against resistance that is varied to maintain high tension throughout range of motion.

Isometric: contractions against an immovable object, static contraction.

Isotonic: contraction against a constant resistance.

Lactic Acid: a fatiguing metabolite of the lactic acid system (anaerobic metabolism) resulting fromincomplete breakdown of carbohydrate.

Lactose: a double sugar composed of glucose and galactose; commonly known as milk sugar.

Lactose Intolerance: inability to digest milk sugar as a result of a lack of the necessary enzyme lactase; ingesting dairy products often results in gastrointestinal distress and diarrhea.

Latent: dormant or concealed; not manifest; potential.

Ligament: tough connective tissue that connects bone to bone.

Lipid: fatty substance; includes triglycerides, phospholipids, and sterols such as cholesterol.

Lipoprotein: lipids in the plasma; they circulate attached to protein.

Low-Density Lipoprotein (LDL): termed "bad" cholesterol; carries cholesterol (much of it synthesized in the liver) to body cells. A high cholesterol usually reflects a high LDL and is a major risk factor for cardiovascular disease.

Legumes: plants of the bean and pea family. The seeds are rich in high-quality protein compared with those of most other plant foods.

Lifestyle Diseases: conditions that may be aggravated by modern lifestyles that include too little exercise, poor diet, excessive drinking and smoking.

Limiting Amino Acid: a term given to the essential amino acid in shortest supply (relative to a body's need) in a given food protein; it therefore limits the body's ability to make its own protein.

Major Mineral: an essential mineral nutrient found in the human body in amounts greater than 5 grams.

Malnutrition: any condition caused by an excess, deficiency, or imbalance of calories or nutrients.

Maltose: a disaccharide composed of two glucose molecules.

Maximal Oxygen Consumption (Uptake): aerobic fitness. A measure of the body's maximal ability to both deliver oxygen to the working muscles and utilize oxygen within working muscles through aerobic metabolism.

Megadose: a dose of ten or more times the amount normally recommended in the RDA. An overdose is an amount high enough to cause toxicity symptoms. Megadoses taken over long periods of time often result in overdose.

Metabolic Fuel: a chemical or food used for energy production; a protein, carbohydrate or fat.

Metabolism: the sum total of the chemical changes or reactions occurring in the body.

Minerals: small, naturally occurring inorganic, chemical elements; the minerals serve as structural components and in many vital processes in the body.

Mitochondria: tiny organelle within cells; site of all oxidative (aerobic) energy production.

Moderation: the attribute of a diet that provides no unwanted constituent in excess.

Monoglyceride: one of the products of digestion of lipids; a glycerol molecule with one fatty acid attached to it.

Monosaccharide: a single sugar from which other carbohydrates are formed; primarily glucose, fructose and galactose.

Monounsaturated Fat: a triglyceride in which one or more of the fatty acids is monounsaturated, found in olive and canola oils.

Monounsaturated Fatty Acid: a fatty acid containing one point of unsaturation.

Mortality: the rate of deaths caused by specific disease within a specific population.

Muscle Fiber Types: fast-twitch fibers are fast contracting, produce large amounts of force, but relatively fast to fatigue; slow-twitch fibers contract somewhat slower, with less force, but are fatigue resistant.

Muscular Fitness: the strength, muscular endurance, and flexibility needed to carry out daily tasks and avoid injury.

Muscle Strain: muscle injury resulting from overexertion or trauma and involving overstretching or tearing of muscle fibers.

Natural Food: one that has been altered as little as possible from the original farm-grown state. As used on labels, this term may misleadingly imply unusual power to promote health; it has no legal definition.

Natural Sweetener: a term without a legal definition; refers to any sugar or sweetener other than refined table sugar—sucrose.

Negative Energy Balance: less energy is consumed than expended and body weight decreases.

Nonheme Iron: the iron found in plant foods.

Nutrient Dense: refers to a food that supplies large amounts of nutrients relative to the number of calories it contains. The higher the level of nutrients and the fewer the number of calories the more nutrient dense the food.

Nutrients: substances obtained from food and used in the body to promote growth, maintenance, and repair.

Nutrition: food, vitamins, minerals, and other nutrients that are ingested and assimilated into the body.

Obesity: condition characterized by abnormally high proportion of body fat.

Oils: lipids that are liquid at room temperature.

Organic: of, related to, or containing carbon compounds.

Osteoporosis: a disease in which bones become porous and fragile.

Overload: an extra physical demand placed on the body. A principle of training is that for a body system to improve, its workload must be increased by increments over time.

Overnutrition: calorie or nutrient overconsumption severe enough to cause disease or increased risk of disease; a form of malnutrition.

Overtraining: excess training that leads to staleness, injury, or illness.

Overweight: conventionally defined as weight between 10 percent and 20 percent above the desirable weight for height.

Oxidized LDL-Cholesterol: the cholesterol in LDLs that is attacked (oxidized) by reactive oxygen molecules inside the walls of the arteries which are deposited in arterial plaque.

Oxygen Uptake: oxygen used in oxidative (aerobic) metabolism.

Perceived Exertion: subjective estimate of exercise difficulty.

Phospholipid: lipid containing phosphorous.

Phytochemicals: chemicals found in plants that are not nutrients but that appear to help fight diseases such as cancer. Phyto = plant.

Polyunsaturated Fat: a triglyceride in which one or more of the fatty acids is polyunsaturated.

Polyunsaturated Fatty Acid: a fatty acid in which two or more points of unsaturated occur.

Positive Energy Balance: more energy is consumed than expended and body weight increases.

Protein Digestibility-Corrected Amino Acid Score (PDCAAS): a measure of protein quality; the PDCAAS takes into account both the amino acid balance of a food and its digestibility.

Protein Quality: a measure of the essential amino acid content of a protein relative to the essential amino acid needs of the body.

Proteins: compounds composed of atoms of carbon, hydrogen, oxygen, and nitrogen arranged as strands of amino acids. Some amino acids also contain atoms of sulfur.

Provitamin: a substance the body can use to form a vitamin. Sometimes referred to as a precursor.

Recommended Nutrient Allowances (RDA): a set of daily nutrient and calorie consumption levels intended to meet the nutritional needs of virtually all healthy people living in the United States. The RDAs are recommendations and individual requirements may vary based of age, health status, activity, and exercise levels.

Recommended Daily Intakes (RDI): a table devised in 1968 listing one suggested intake for vitamins, minerals, and other nutrients. The RDI are not intended as nutritional goals that everyone should meet. Rather they are for use on food labels to help people get an idea of the amount of nutrients a serving of the product contributes to the diet. The RDI were known as the U.S. Recommended Daily Allowances (U.S. RDA) until the food labels were revamped in 1993.

Refined: refers to the process by which the course parts of food products are removed. For example, the refining of wheat into flour involves removing three of the four parts of the kernel—the chaff, bran, and germ—leaving only the ectosperm (starch, with only little protein or fiber).

Repetition Maximum (RM): the maximal load that a muscle or muscle group can lift in a given number of repetitions, with correct form, before fatiguing. For example, an eight-RM load is the maximum load that can be lifted with proper form eight times.

Requirement: the minimum amount of a nutrient in the diet that will prevent the development of deficiency symptoms.

Risk: the harm a substance may confer. Scientists estimate risk by assessing the amount of a chemical that each person in a population might consume over time, also called exposure, and by considering how toxic the substance might be.

Risk Factor: predisposing condition; factor that puts one at a higher than usual risk for developing a disease. Heredity or lifestyle factors that help determine the likelihood of disease.

Saccharin: a zero-calorie sweetener discovered in 1879 and used in the United States since the turn of the century. A possible link to bladder cancer led to saccharin's being banned as a food additive in Canada, although it is available there as a tabletop sweetener; it is used with a warning label in the United States.

Salt: a pair of charged mineral ions, most commonly sodium ($Na+$) and chloride ($Cl-$), that are associated together.

Salt Sensitive: the tendency for blood pressure to rise in proportion to salt consumption that certain people seem to have, making up only 20 percent of all hypertensive individuals.

Satiety: the feeling of fullness or satisfaction that people feel after meals.

Saturated Fatty Acid: a fatty acid carrying the maximum possible number of hydrogen atoms, having no points of unsaturation. A saturated fat is one that is made up primarily of saturated fatty acids, which are associated with an elevated blood cholesterol and increased risk of disease.

Serving: the amount of food a person might eat, usually much larger than a serving.

Set: in an interval-training program, a group of work and relief intervals. In weight lifting, the number of repetitions performed consecutively without resting.

Set-Point Theory: the theory that the body tends to maintain a certain weight by adjusting hunger, appetite, and food intake on the one hand and metabolism (energy output) on the other so that a person's conscious efforts to alter weight may be foiled.

Simple Carbohydrates: (sugars) the simple sugars, monosaccharides and the pairs of sugars, disaccharides, linked together.

Soluble Fiber: includes the fiber types called pectin, gums, and mucilages; soluble fibers either dissolve or swell when placed in water. Soluble fibers are found in fruits, oats and oat products and are associated with lowered blood cholesterol and blood insulin levels.

Somatotype: body types; ectomorph is linear or thin, mesomorph is muscular, and endomorph is fat.

Specificity: a principle of training that states that the type of training undertaken must relate to the desired results—you get what you train for.

Starch: a plant polysaccharide composed of glucose, digestible by human beings.

Sterols: one of the three main classes of lipids; a lipid with a structure similar to cholesterol.

Strength: the ability of muscles to work against resistance.

Strength (Resistance) Training: contracting muscles against resistance to enhance muscle strength, power, endurance or size.

Stress: any threat, be it physical or psychological, to a person's well-being.

Subcutaneous Fat: fat deposits and storage beneath the skin.

Sucrose: a disaccharide composed of fructose and glucose.

Target Heart Rate: the heartbeat rate that will achieve a cardiovascular conditioning effect for a given person. Calculated by multiplying 65 percent, for the lower limit, and 90 percent, for the upper limit by the person's maximal predicted heart rate. Maximal heart rate is calculated by subtracting one's age from 220; units are in beats per minute.

Tendon: tough connective tissue that connects muscle to bone.

Thermoregulation: the regulation of the body's temperature.

Tonus: muscle firmness in absence of a voluntary contraction.

Toxicity: the ability of a substance to harm living organisms. All substances are toxic if present in high enough concentrations.

Trace Mineral: an essential mineral found in the human body in amounts of less than 5 grams.

Training: a program of exercise designed to improve the skills and increase the energy capacities of an athlete for a particular event.

Training Stimulus: the type of exercise that elicits the desired adaptation to training.

Training Zone: the heart rate zone within which training is likely to produce the desired effect.

Trans-Fatty Acid: a type of fatty acid created when an unsaturated fat is hydrogenated. Found primarily in margarines, shortening, commercial frying fats, and baked goods, trans fatty acids have been implicated in preliminary research as culprits in heart disease.

Triglycerides: the major class of dietary lipids, including fats and oils. A triglyceride is made up of three units known as fatty acids and one unit called glycerol.

Underweight: weight 10 percent or more below the desirable weight for height.

Unsaturated Fatty Acid: a fatty acid in which one or more points of unsaturation occur; either monounsaturated or polyunsaturated. An unsaturated fat is a triglyceride in which one or more of the fatty acids in unsaturated.

Vitamin: a potent, indispensable compound that performs various bodily functions that promote growth and reproduction and maintain health. Vitamins are organic, meaning that they contain or are related to carbon compounds. Contrary to popular belief, vitamins do not supply energy or calories.

Very-Low-Density Lipoprotein: carries fats, primarily triglycerides, packaged or made by the liver to various tissues of the body.

Weight Training: progressive resistance exercise using weight for resistance.

Wellness: a conscious and deliberate approach to an advanced state of physiological, psychological, and spiritual health.

Whole Food: a food that is altered as little as possible from the plant or animal tissue from which it was taken, such as beets, milk, or oats.

Work Capacity: the ability to achieve work goals without undue fatigue.

Index

Page numbers in *italics* indicate figures; those in **bold** indicate charts.

About the Author

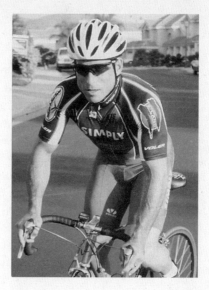

Eric Sternlicht, Ph.D., is that rare breed of expert who is as at home in the field as he is in a lab. A distinguished scientist, researcher, and athlete, he weaves nutrition, aerobic exercise, anaerobic exercise, and recovery into an integrated, realistic system. In an age of increasing confusion, he is a beacon of common sense, logic, and integrity.

A lifelong athlete, Sternlicht has been skiing since he was four, swam on national-caliber swim teams in his youth, and walked away from a professional freestyle ski career when he was eighteen in favor of college. There, while studying physiology at UCLA, he added bodybuilding to his roster of competitive sports, trained with soon-to-be Mr. America, Tony Pearson, and in 1980, won the first bodybuilding competition he ever entered, the Collegiate Mr. America. He competed for the next eight years in state and regional competitions. "I was studying for my master's and doctorate degrees, and welcomed the escape the training provided."

In 1985, while still working on his Ph.D., he started his own consulting business, Simply Fit. His combination of academic credentials and his look helped him become one of Hollywood's most sought-after trainers and consultants, giving him the chance to work with entertainers such as Lou Ferrigno, Deborah Shelton, and Clint Eastwood.

Although he relocated to Orange County in 1989, he continued to consult for professional athletes, including cyclists, runners, and triathletes, elite athletes from UCLA and Purdue, entertainers, and corporations such as Disney, Sony, and ESPN. Then, in 1991, Reebok hired him to develop the

Slide Reebok Training Program, including the training guidelines and all the educational materials involved in the product launch, such as the workout, training manuals, videos, and collateral materials. In the rollout, he lectured extensively throughout America and the world. Throughout the three-year duration of this project, Sternlicht continued to carry a full teaching load at two colleges, UCLA and Occidental College in Los Angeles; and appeared as an expert guest consultant on ESPN's *Body Shaping*.

By then he had also become a competitive cyclist. In the past ten years, he started the Simply Fit Cycling Team, which has grown from a handful of friends to over two hundred members nationwide, including several former Olympians and a number of national and world champions. He himself has won the California State Time Trial Championships four times and placed second in the 1999 Masters National Championships, and won the 2001 Masters National Championships.

The same time he was besting his cycling competition, he was experiencing his biggest professional win as well. His dual expertise in nutrition and training prompted the Swiss cosmetic company, Arbonne International, to ask him to develop a top-flight series of supplements and foods devoted specifically toward weight management, fitness, and sports nutrition. In addition to formulating the products, he developed all the educational materials supporting the launch. Here at last was a chance to put all the research and information to practical use, and tailor-make products that enabled people to train for optimal performance.

Now that the research has been done, Sternlicht wants to teach the general public how to use sports nutrition to train and live better. Given his natural ability to not just understand the science but make it accessible, it is the logical next move in an already extraordinary career.